Dasgupta's
Recent Advances in
Obstetrics and Gynecology

AF520944

Dasgupta's

Recent Advances in Obstetrics and Gynecology

Volume 14

Editor

Nandita Palshetkar

MD FCPS FICOG FRCOG (UK)

Professor Emeritus

Department of Obstetrics and Gynecology

DY Patil School of Medicine

Navi Mumbai, Maharashtra, India

Infertility Specialist, Lilavati Hospital IVF Center, Mumbai

Founder and Medical Director, Bloom IVF and BAUFICI Genetics

President, Indian Society for Assisted Reproduction (2022–2024)

President, Association of Maharashtra Obstetric and Gynaecological Societies (2020–2022)

Past President, FOGSI, IAGE, MOGS and MSR

Co-Editors

Pratik Tambe

MD FICOG FICRM FICMCH FIAOG

ART Consultant and Gynecological Endoscopic Surgeon

Ashirwad IVF, Mumbai, Maharashtra, India

Governing Council Member, ICOG and ICRM

Managing Committee Member, ISAR, MOGS, MSR

Rohan Palshetkar

MS (Obs & Gyne) FRM BDRME ADRME

ART Consultant and Endoscopic Surgeon

Professor

Department of Reproductive Medicine

DY Patil Medical College

Unit Head

DY Patil Bloom IVF and Opera House Bloom IVF

Mumbai, Maharashtra, India

JAYPEE

JAYPEE BROTHERS MEDICAL PUBLISHERS

The Health Sciences Publisher

New Delhi | London

Jaypee Brothers Medical Publishers (P) Ltd

Headquarters

EMCA House, 23/23-B
Ansari Road, Daryaganj
New Delhi 110 002, India
Landline: +91-11-23272143, +91-11-23272703
+91-11-23282021, +91-11-23245672
e-mail: jaypee@jaypeebrothers.com

Corporate Office

4838/24, Ansari Road, Daryaganj
New Delhi 110 002, India
Phone: +91-11-43574357
Fax: +91-11-43574314
e-mail: jaypee@jaypeebrothers.com

Overseas Office

JP Medical Ltd.
83, Victoria Street, London
SW1H 0HW (UK)
Phone: +44-20 3170 8910
e-mail: info@jpmedpub.com

EU GPSR Authorised Representative

Logos Europe, 9 rue Nicolas Poussin
17000, La Rochelle, France
Phone: +33 (0) 6 67 93 73 78
e-mail: contact@logoseurope.eu

Website: www.jaypeebrothers.com
Website: www.jaypeedigital.com

© 2025, Jaypee Brothers Medical Publishers

The views and opinions expressed in this book are solely those of the original contributor(s)/author(s) and do not necessarily represent those of editor(s) or publisher of the book.

All rights reserved. No part of this publication may be reproduced, stored or transmitted in any form or by any means, electronic, mechanical, photocopying, recording or otherwise, without the prior permission in writing of the publishers.

All brand names and product names used in this book are trade names, service marks, trademarks or registered trademarks of their respective owners. The publisher is not associated with any product or vendor mentioned in this book.

Medical knowledge and practice change constantly. This book is designed to provide accurate, authoritative information about the subject matter in question. However, readers are advised to check the most current information available on procedures included and check information from the manufacturer of each product to be administered, to verify the recommended dose, formula, method and duration of administration, adverse effects and contraindications. It is the responsibility of the practitioner to take all appropriate safety precautions. Neither the publisher nor the author(s)/editor(s) assume any liability for any injury and/or damage to persons or property arising from or related to use of material in this book.

This book is sold on the understanding that the publisher is not engaged in providing professional medical services. If such advice or services are required, the services of a competent medical professional should be sought.

Every effort has been made where necessary to contact holders of copyright to obtain permission to reproduce copyright material. If any have been inadvertently overlooked, the publisher will be pleased to make the necessary arrangements at the first opportunity.

Inquiries for bulk sales may be solicited at: jaypee@jaypeebrothers.com

Dasgupta's Recent Advances in Obstetrics and Gynecology (Volume 14)

First Edition: **2025**

ISBN: 978-93-5696-766-3

Printed and bound at Sterling Graphics Pvt. Ltd. Manesar

Dedicated to

Our mentors, teachers, and our patients

Contributors

Abha Rani Sinha MBBS DGO MS
Principal and Professor
Department of Obstetrics and Gynecology
Sri Krishna Medical College
Muzaffarpur, Bihar, India

Aditya Rajiv Nimbkar
MS (Obs & Gyne) DNB MBBS
Assistant Professor
Department of Obstetrics and Gynecology
Seth GS Medical College and KEM Hospital
Mumbai, Maharashtra, India

Annith Kumar VM MS MRCOG
Scientific Director
Promise Fertility Center
Assistant Professor
Department of Obstetrics and Gynecology
Tagore Medical College
Chennai, Tamil Nadu, India

Anupama Bahadur DNB MNAMS
Professor and Unit Head
Department of Obstetrics and Gynecology
All India Institute of Medical Sciences
Rishikesh, Uttarakhand, India

Athulya Shajan
MBBS MS (Obs & Gyne)
Consultant Gynecologist
Department of Reproductive Medicine and Surgery
CIMAR—the Women's Hospital
Thrissur, Kerala, India

Ayushi Heda
MD DNB MCh (Gynae-Oncology)
Senior Resident
Department of Obstetrics and Gynecology
All India Institute of Medical Sciences
Rishikesh, Uttarakhand, India

Bhagyalaxmi Nayak MD PhD
Professor and Head
Department of Gynecologic Oncology
Acharya Harihar Postgraduate Institute of Oncology
Cuttack, Odisha, India

Charmila Ayyavoo
MD DGO DFP FICOG PGDCR
Director, Aditi Hospital
Assistant Professor
Department of Obstetrics and Gynecology
Dhanalakshmi Srinivasan Medical College and Hospital
Perambalur, Tamil Nadu, India

Deepali Prakash Kale
MBBS DGO FCPS DNB FMAS
Associate Professor
Department of Obstetrics and Gynecology
Seth GS Medical College and Nowrosjee Wadia Maternity Hospital
Mumbai, Maharashtra, India

Geetendra Sharma
MD LLB (Gold Medalist)
Medicolegal Consultant
B&S Medicolegal Consultancies
Vice President, FOGSI (2022–2023)

Girija Wagh
MD FICOG Dip Endoscopy FICS
Professor and Head
Department of Obstetrics and Gynecology
Bharati Vidyapeeth University Medical College, Pune, Maharashtra, India
Director, Primrose Wellness and Care
Consultant
Apollo Spectra Hospitals, Pune
Vice President, FOGSI

Gorakh G Mandrupkar
MBBS DGO FCPS FICOG MSc
IVF Consultant
Department of Reproductive Medicine
Mandrupkar Clinic
Sangli, Maharashtra, India

HP Pattnaik MD FICOG FICMCH
Senior Consultant (Obstetrics and Gynecology) and Endoscopic Surgeon
Health Line Nursing Home
Cuttack, Odisha, India
Former Director of Health Services and Director of Public Health, Odisha
Former Special Secretary, Odisha
Vice President, FOGSI 2009
President, IMS 2015
Secretary General, SOVSI

Hrishikesh D Pai
MD FRCOG (UK-HON) FCPS FICOG MSc (USA)
Founder and Medical Director
Bloom IVF Group, Lilavati Hospital IVF Center, Mumbai, Maharashtra, India
Consultant Gynecologist
Lilavati Hospital IVF Center, Mumbai and Fortis Hospital Bloom IVF Centre Delhi and Chandigarh
Professor
Department of Reproductive Medicine
DY Patil University, Navi Mumbai
Immediate Past President, FOGSI (2022–2023)
Trustee, FIGO Asia Oceania (2023–2025)
Chief Administrator
FOGSI Manyata Project
Postgraduate Teacher for MD and DNB Courses (1991–2018)

Jash Tank MBBS
Student, III/II MBBS
Padmashree Dr DY Patil University
School of Medicine
Mumbai, Maharashtra, India

Kanchan Prasad
MS (Obs & Gyne) FICOG FIAOG FRM FMAS
Professor
Department of Obstetrics and Gynecology
Teerthanker Mahaveer Medical College and Research Centre
Moradabad, Uttar Pradesh, India

Karishma Kirti
MBBS MS (General surgery) MCh Principles of Breast Oncoplasty (UK)
Consultant and Assistant Professor
Department of Surgical Oncology
Jaslok Hospital and Research Centre
Mumbai, Maharashtra, India
HBNI Breast Oncology Fellowship (Tata Memorial Hospital)
European Society of Surgical Oncology Fellowship (ESSO-FEBS)
Visiting Fellowship in Breast Oncoplasty, institut du sein (France)

Keshav Malhotra MBBS MCE FICRM
Embryologist and Lab Director
Department of Embrylogy
Rainbow IVF, Agra, Uttar Pradesh, India

Lila Vyas MBBS MS
Director, HOPE Hospital
Senior Consultant
Department of Obstetrics and Gynecology
Vyas Clinic, Cocoon Hospital
Jaipur, Rajasthan, India
Former Senior Professor
SMS Medical College, Jaipur
Vice President, FOGSI 2018

Mahesh Gupta MD (Gyne)
Proprietor and Director
Matis Multispeciality Hospital
Ahmedabad, Gujarat, India

Manila Kaushal
MS DNB FRCOG MNAMS FICOG
Professor
Department of Obstetrics and Gynecology
Mahi Women's Clinic and Surgical Center
Indore, Madhya Pradesh, India

Muralidhar V Pai
MBBS DGO MD (Obs & Gyne) FRCOG FICOG FKCOG FICMCH
Dean
Department of Obstetrics and Gynecology
Sikkim Manipal Institute of Medical Sciences
Sikkim Manipal University
Gangtok, Sikkim, India

N Sanjeeva Reddy MD DGO
Professor
Department of Reproductive Medicine and Surgery
Sri Ramachandra Institute of Higher Education and Research (Deemed to be University)
Chennai, Tamil Nadu, India

Namrata Ray Ohri
MBBS MS (Obs & Gyne)
Consultant
Department of Obstetrics and Gynecology
New Life Hospital and Healthcare Pvt Ltd, Varanasi, Uttar Pradesh, India

Nandita Palshetkar
MD FCPS FICOG FRCOG (UK)
Professor Emeritus
Department of Obstetrics and Gynecology
DY Patil School of Medicine
Navi Mumbai, Maharashtra, India
Infertility Specialist, Lilavati Hospital IVF Center, Mumbai
Founder and Medical Director
Bloom IVF and BAUFICI Genetics
President, Indian Society for Assisted Reproduction (2022–2024)
President, Association of Maharashtra Obstetric and Gynaecological Societies (2020–2022)
Past President, FOGSI, IAGE, MOGS and MSR

Neelam Ohri MBBS MS (Obs & Gyne)
Medical Director
Department of Obstetrics and Gynecology
New Life Hospital and Healthcare Pvt Ltd
Varanasi, Uttar Pradesh, India

Neharika Malhotra
MD (Obs & Gyne, Gold Medalist)
DRM (Germany) FICOG
Consultant
Department of Obstetrics and Gynecology
Ujala Cygnus Rainbow Hospital and Rainbow IVF
Agra, Uttar Pradesh, India

Nita S Nair
MBBS DNB (Gen Surg) MRCS (Ed)
MCh (Surg Onco)
Consultant Surgeon
Department of Surgical Oncology
Apollo Cancer Centre
Navi Mumbai, Maharashtra, India

Pratik Tambe
MD FICOG FICRM FICMCH FIAOG
ART Consultant and Gynecological Endoscopic Surgeon
Ashirwad IVF
Mumbai, Maharashtra, India
Governing Council Member
ICOG and ICRM
Managing Committee Member
ISAR, MOGS, MSR
Past Chair, FOGSI Endocrinology Committee (2017–2019)
Past Chair, AMOGS Endocrinology Committee (2020–2024)

Priya Gupta MBBS MS
Director
Maa & Me Maternity Hospital and Infertility Centre
Senior Consultant
Department of Obstetrics and Gynecology
Kota Heart Institute and Shriji Hospital
Kota, Rajasthan, India

Priyankur Roy
MBBS MS (OBG) DRM FAGE
Senior Consultant Gynecologist
Department of Reproductive Medicine and Surgery
Roy's Clinic and Multispeciality Hospital
Siliguri, West Bengal, India

Radha Vembu MBBS DGO DNB PhD
Professor and Head
Department of Reproductive Medicine and Surgery
Sri Ramachandra Institute of Higher Education and Research
(Deemed to be University)
Chennai, Tamil Nadu, India

Riddhi Desai
MS FICOG PGDMLS Dip Endoscopy (Pune, USA)
Dip Office Hysteroscopy (Italy) CIMP
Consultant
Department of Obstetrics and Gynecology
Advanced Multispeciality Hospital
Mumbai, Maharashtra, India

Rohan Palshetkar
MS (Obs & Gyne) FRM BDRME ADRME
ART Consultant and Endoscopic Surgeon
Professor
Department of Reproductive Medicine
DY Patil Medical College
Unit Head
DY Patil Bloom IVF and Opera House Bloom IVF
Mumbai, Maharashtra, India

Roza Olyai
MS FICMCH FICOG
HoD
Department of Obstetrics and Gynecology
Olyai Hospital
Gwalior, Madhya Pradesh, India
President, Gwalior Obstetrics and Gynecological Society

Sakshi Heda MD DNB
Senior Resident
Department of Obstetrics and Gynecology
All India Institute of Medical Sciences
Rishikesh, Uttarakhand, India

Shilpa Nitin Chaudhari
MD (Obs & Gyne)
Professor
Department of Obstetrics and Gynecology
Smt Kashibai Navale Medical College and General Hospital
Pune, Maharashtra, India

Sonali Tank MD (Paediatrics)
Consultant Pediatrician and Neonatologist
The Ashwini Clinic
Mumbai, Maharashtra, India

Sridevi Murali-Nanavati
MBBS MS (Gen Surg) HBNI Breast Oncology Fellowship (Tata Memorial Hospital) FEBS CEBS
Associate Consultant
Department of Breast Oncology
Nanavati Max Super Specialty Hospital
Mumbai, Maharashtra, India

Suchitra Pandit MD DNB FICOG BPharm
Consultant
Department of Obstetrics and Gynecology
Surya Hospital
Mumbai, Maharashtra, India

Suyesha Khanijao MBBS DNB
Director
IVF Expert, Gynecologist, Obstetrician and Cosmetic Gynecologist
Angel's Hope IVF
Sawan Neelu Angel's Hospital
New Delhi, India

Swati Bhargava MS (Obs & Gyne)
Consultant
Former Associate Professor
MGM Medical College
Indore, Madhya Pradesh, India

Vidya Thobbi MD FICOG
Professor
Department of Obstetrics and Gynecology
Alameen Medical College
Vijayapur, Karnataka, India

Vinita Kumari MBBS MS
Associate Professor
Department of Obstetrics and Gynecology
Nalanda Medical College
Patna, Bihar, India

Preface

Respected colleagues and dear friends,

It is with immense pride that we bring to you this 14th edition of *Dasgupta's Recent Advances in Obstetrics and Gynecology*. This series is aimed at postgraduate students who need a single volume covering all the latest advances in our field.

Our greatest weakness lies in giving up. The most certain way to succeed is always to try just one more time. ***–Thomas A Edison***

The postgraduate curriculum has undergone several changes over the past few decades. There is greater emphasis on modern methodology of management incorporating the latest algorithms and the newest guidelines which are being published regularly. Hence, we continue the excellent series of Dasgupta's Recent Advances in this 14th edition with clinically relevant topics which are authored by some of the seniormost and most sought-after teachers in the country.

With the enormous pressure of clinical work, postgraduate students often do not have much time to research topics, hunt for references, and sift through the mountains of published evidence to imbibe the most relevant information which is essential for them during the examinations. Each of the chapters in this book is therefore a crash course on the subject and will serve the reader well by focusing on traditional concepts as well as the most modern updated evidence on the issues at hand.

We hope that this book will be a useful compendium for postgraduate students and readers who wish to keep themselves updated with the latest evidence on the topics which we have covered. The chapters have been authored in a simple, easy to understand, and concise fashion.

We welcome your feedback on this volume and suggestions for future topics which you may wish to see covered.

Yours sincerely,

Nandita Palshetkar
Pratik Tambe
Rohan Palshetkar

Preface

Acknowledgments

The editors would like to acknowledge the efforts of all the authors and coauthors in the preparation of the manuscript, revision of their chapters, and for being in constant communication with us despite their busy schedules.

We are extremely thankful to Shri Jitendar P Vij (Group Chairman), Ms Chetna Malhotra (Senior Director—Professional Publishing, Marketing, and Business Development), and Pragati Singh (Development Editor) of M/s Jaypee Brothers Medical Publishers (P) Ltd, New Delhi, India, for their hard work, coordination, and support toward the publication of this book.

Contents

CHAPTER 1 Neonatal Resuscitation

Sonali Tank, Jash Tank

INTRODUCTION

The first hour after birth has a major influence on the survival, future health, and well-being of a newborn. Nearly 85% of term newborns begin breathing within 30 seconds after birth, 10% respond to drying and stimulation, and 1% need extensive resuscitation.[1,2] Birth asphyxia accounts for 23% of neonatal deaths occurring worldwide.[3] It contributes to one-fifth of all neonatal deaths in India.[2]

INTRAUTERINE TO EXTRAUTERINE TRANSITION[1]

- *Before birth,* fetal lungs are filled with fluid.
- *After birth,* three major changes occur:
  1. As the baby cries, fluid is absorbed from the alveoli and the lungs fill with air.
  2. This relaxes the constricted pulmonary vessels, blood flows to the lungs, and oxygen is absorbed.
  3. Once the cord is clamped, oxygenated blood reaches the baby's heart and brain. Though this occurs within a few minutes of birth, it is shown that it may take up to 10 minutes to achieve an oxygen saturation of 90% or more.[4] The entire process may not be completed for hours to days.

KEY TO SUCCESSFUL RESUSCITATION

Anticipation, preparation, evaluation, and prompt measures are critical for successful resuscitation. Each delivery should have one person who is capable of initiating resuscitation, giving positive-pressure ventilation, chest compressions (CCs), intubation, and medications.[4,5]

Delivery Room Preparation

Equipment must be clean, checked before each delivery, and be of the correct size.

- Mucus extractor and suction catheter should discarded after use.
- If an electrical suction machine is used, the pressure should not exceed a negative pressure of 100 mm Hg.
- Switch on the radiant warmer 20 minutes before delivery, close the windows, and switch off the fan.
- Test the function of the bag and mask and ensure the laryngoscope is working.

Neonatal Resuscitation Program Algorithm[1]

The Neonatal Resuscitation Program (NRP) algorithm **(Flowchart 1)** describes steps to follow to evaluate and resuscitate a newborn.

Flowchart 1: NRP algorithm.

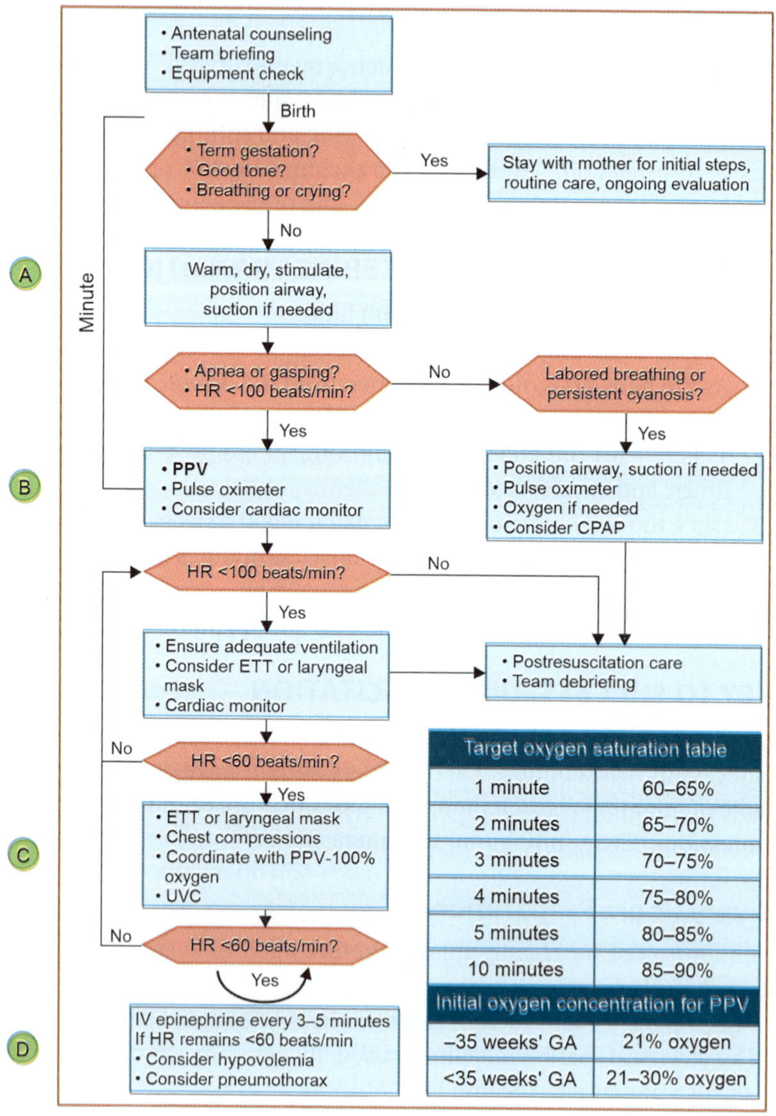

Target oxygen saturation table	
1 minute	60–65%
2 minutes	65–70%
3 minutes	70–75%
4 minutes	75–80%
5 minutes	80–85%
10 minutes	85–90%
Initial oxygen concentration for PPV	
–35 weeks' GA	21% oxygen
<35 weeks' GA	21–30% oxygen

(CPAP: continuous positive airway pressure; ETT: endotracheal tube; GA: gestational age; HR: heart rate; IV: intravenous; NRP: neonatal resuscitation program; PPV: positive pressure ventilation; UVC: umbilical venous catheter)

In **Flowchart 1**, hexagons indicate assessments and rectangles show actions required. Ensure that you perform the steps of each block before moving on to the next.

Questions asked before every birth?[1]

- Expected gestational age?
- Is the amniotic fluid clear?
- Additional risk factors? Knowing the perinatal risk factors will identify more than half of newborns who may need resuscitation **(Box 1)**.
- Umbilical cord management plan?

The ideal time for clamping the cord is the subject of ongoing research. For most vigorous newborns, evidence suggests delaying clamping for 30–60 seconds. Immediate cord clamping is considered where the placental circulation is not intact (placenta previa/vasa previa, abruption, etc.).

BOX 1: Perinatal risk factors increasing the likelihood of neonatal resuscitation.[1]

- *Antepartum risk factors:*
  - Gestational age <36 0/7 weeks
  - Gestational age ≥41 0/7 weeks
  - Preeclampsia or eclampsia
  - Maternal hypertension
  - Multiple gestation
  - Fetal anemia
  - *Polyhydramnios:*
    - Oligohydramnios
    - Fetal hydrops
    - Fetal macrosomia
    - Intrauterine growth restriction
    - Significant fetal malformations or anomalies
  - No prenatal care
- *Intrapartum risk factors:*
  - Forceps or vacuum-assisted delivery
  - Emergency cesarean delivery
  - Breech or other abnormal presentation
  - Abnormal fetal heart rate (HR) pattern
  - *Maternal general anesthesia:*
    - Maternal magnesium therapy
    - Placental abruption
  - *Intrapartum bleeding:*
    - Chorioamnionitis
    - Opioids administered to mother within 4 hours of delivery
  - Shoulder dystocia
  - Meconium-stained amniotic fluid
  - Prolapsed umbilical cord

Evaluating the Newborn After Birth

In the interval between birth and umbilical cord clamping, evaluate the baby to see:

- If they can remain with the mother (term babies) or move to a radiant warmer (preterm babies).
- Check the muscle tone. Healthy-term babies should be active with flexed extremities. Newborns requiring intervention may have flaccid extremities.
- See if the baby is breathing/crying. A vigorous cry indicates strong respiratory effort. If not crying, observe the chest for breathing.

What are the initial steps?[1]

Within 30 seconds of birth:

- *For vigorous, term newborns:*
  - Provide warmth
  - Dry
  - Stimulate
  - Position head and neck
  - Clear secretions if needed
- *For nonvigorous or preterm newborns:* If the answer to any question is "No," bring the baby to a radiant warmer.[6]

Warmth

Place the baby under a radiant warmer to prevent heat loss. Maintain the temperature at 36.5–37.5°C.

Dry

Wet skin increases evaporative heat loss. Gently dry any fluid with a warm towel.

Stimulate

- Drying the baby provides stimulation to initiate breathing. If not, gently rubbing the newborn's back, trunk or extremities may stimulate it.
- Overly vigorous stimulation can cause injury.
- Never shake a baby.

Position

Position the baby on the back with the head and neck neutral or slightly extended, eyes directed straight upward in the "sniffing the morning air position". This opens the airway.

- Avoid hyperextension/flexion of the neck
- You may place a small rolled towel under the baby's shoulders.

If needed, clear airway secretions: Clear the airway if secretions obstruct it, if the baby is not breathing, is gasping, has poor tone, or if you anticipate starting positive pressure ventilation (PPV).

If there are copious secretions coming from the mouth, turn the head to the side. Suction the mouth before the nose so that the baby does not aspirate if the baby gasps when the nose is suctioned.

Vigorous or deep suctioning may injure tissues. Stimulation of the posterior pharynx can produce a vagal response causing bradycardia and apnea.

Evaluation of response: Assess respiration to determine if the baby is responding (should not take more than another 30 seconds).

Baby apneic or gasping?

Proceed directly to PPV, as delaying it beyond the first minute of life worsens the outcome. Ventilation of the baby's lungs is the most important and effective step during neonatal resuscitation.

If the baby is breathing, check the heart rate (HR): If the breathing is effective, the HR should be at least 100 beats/min. If not, *start PPV even if the baby is breathing.* Auscultate along the left side of the chest. Estimate the HR by counting the number of beats in 6 seconds and multiplying by 10.

A pulse oximeter or cardiac monitor may be needed here.

Palpation of pulsations at the umbilical cord base is less accurate and may underestimate the true HR.

Baby has labored breathing or persistently low oxygen?

Consider a trial of continuous positive airway pressure (CPAP) or PPV.

In the Case of Meconium-stained Amniotic Fluid

The presence of meconium may indicate fetal distress and increase the risk of needing resuscitation.

- If the baby is vigorous and has good respiratory effort and muscle tone—follow the initial steps of newborn care.
- If the baby is nonvigorous, has depressed respiration or poor muscle tone, bring the baby to the warmer, perform the initial steps, and clear secretions.
- In case the baby is not breathing or breathing but HR is <100 beats/min, proceed with PPV.

ASSISTED VENTILATION DEVICES[1,7,8] (FIGS. 1A TO C)

Free-flow Oxygen

Free-flow oxygen is given when the pulse oximeter reading remains below the target range. It is given by holding the oxygen tubing close to the baby's mouth and nose (cupping the hand increases O_2 concentration). Adjust the flow meter to 10 L/min. Start with 30% and adjust the FiO_2 to maintain saturation within the target range.

Three types of devices are commonly used:

1. *Self-inflating bag (Ambu bag):* This is found commonly in the delivery room. It is easier to use as it reinflates after being squeezed. It has a pressure release valve (which makes overinflation less likely) and does not require a compressed gas source. When used with a mask forming a tight seal and an oxygen reservoir, it delivers 90–100% oxygen. If not attached to an oxygen source, the bag fills by drawing in room air (21% oxygen).
2. *Flow-inflating bag* (used by anesthetists) can deliver 100% oxygen but requires a compressed gas source and a pressure gauge. It takes practice to use effectively. As there is no safety valve, the degree of chest movement has to be watched *each* time to prevent over/under-inflation of the lungs.
3. *T-piece resuscitator:* It is a mechanical device that uses valves to regulate the flow of compressed gas received by the patient. It requires a compressed gas source. A breath is delivered by using a finger to alternately occlude and release a gas escape opening on the top of the T-piece cap.

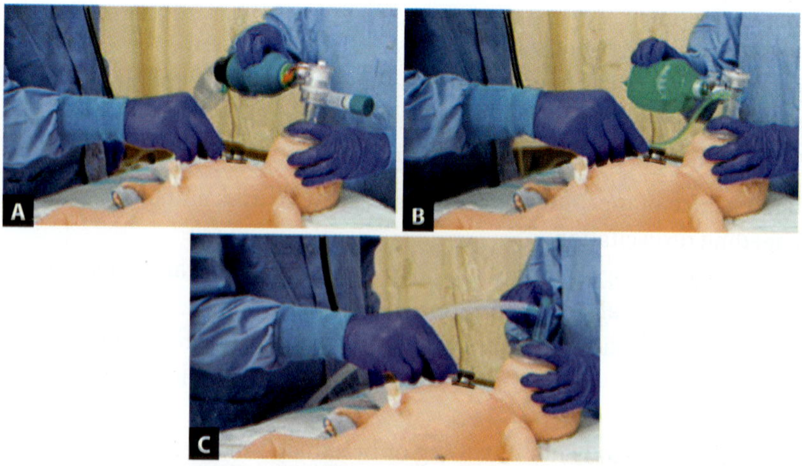

Figs. 1A to C: Positive pressure ventilation. (A) Self-inflating bag; (B) Flow-inflating bag; (C) T-piece resuscitator.

INDICATIONS OF POSITIVE PRESSURE VENTILATION

If the baby is not breathing/apneic, is gasping, or if the HR is <100 beats/min. When indicated, it should be started within 1 minute of birth.

A trial may also be given if the baby is breathing, HR is ≥100 beats/min, but O_2 saturation cannot be maintained in the target range despite free-flow O_2 or CPAP.

Preparation

Position

The person responsible for positioning the airway and holding the mask stands at the baby's head so that the other team members can stand at the side of the bed to help in resuscitation. The baby's head and neck should be positioned in the midline, in a sniffing position.

Selection of Mask

The rim of the mask should cover the tip of the chin, mouth, and nose but not the eyes. If the mask is large, it may cause eye damage and will not seal well. If small, it will not cover the mouth and nose and may occlude the nose.

Shape

It should be cushioned, round or anatomically shaped, be of soft flexible material, and form a good seal.

Method

Begin by cupping the chin in the bottom of the anatomic mask and then bring the mask over the mouth and nose, making sure the bottom is resting on the chin and the head is in a sniffing position. An airtight seal between the rim of the mask and the face is necessary to achieve the pressure to inflate the lungs. The mask usually is held on the face with the thumb, index, and/or middle finger encircling the rim in the shape of the letter "C" while the ring and fifth fingers bring the chin forward to maintain a patent airway.

Oxygen Concentration

Studies have shown that resuscitation starting with 21% O_2 in term and late preterm newborns and 21–30% in preterms is just as effective as 100% oxygen.[9]

Ventilation Rate

Breaths should be given at a rate of 40–60/min. Use the rhythm—breathe, two, three; breathe, two, three. Say "breathe" as you squeeze the bag and release when you say "two, three."

Pressure

For gas exchange to occur after birth, the fetal lung fluid must be replaced with air. Use just enough pressure to inflate the lungs and increase saturation. Once the lungs are inflated, watch for a gentle rise and fall of the chest with each breath. Full-term babies may require a higher pressure for the first few breaths.

The most important indicator of successful PPV is rising HR. It should increase within 15 seconds and be >100 beats/min in 30 seconds.[3,10]

If the HR is increasing after 15 seconds, continue PPV, and reassess after 30 seconds. If 100 beats/min or more, continue ventilating till the HR remains above 100 beats/min. Then, gradually reduce the rate and stop PPV once the baby has sustained spontaneous breathing.

If the HR is not increasing in the first 15 seconds, ask the assistant if the chest is moving. If yes, continue PPV while you monitor the ventilation technique.

If the chest is not moving, you may not be ventilating the lungs. Perform the *ventilation corrective steps* as described until chest movement is achieved.

Ventilation corrective steps (1) are a series of adjustments to be made if the baby's HR is not improving and the chest is not moving.

Use the mnemonic MR. SOPA to remember the steps in order.

M: Mask adjustment
R: Reposition head and neck
S: Suction mouth and nose
O: Open the mouth
P: Pressure increase
A: Alternative airway

Perform the steps sequentially until chest movements with assisted breaths are achieved.

If the HR is 60–100 beats/min, continue PPV as long as there is steady improvement. If not already done, insert an endotracheal tube.

If the HR is <60 beats/min despite using ventilation corrective steps but chest movement is there, begin CCs.

CPAP: Considered if the baby is breathing spontaneously and has an HR of at least 100 beats/min but has labored or grunting respiration.

It helps maintain pressure within the lungs of a *spontaneously breathing* baby. It keeps the lungs slightly inflated at all times. It also helps preterm babies whose lungs are surfactant deficient causing the alveoli to collapse at the end of each exhalation. When CPAP is provided, the baby does not have to work as hard to inflate the lungs. Early use in preterm newborns may avoid the need for intubation and mechanical ventilation.

It is administered by making a seal between the baby's face and a mask attached to either a T-piece resuscitator or a flow-inflating bag. It *cannot* be administered with a self-inflating bag. The desired CPAP is achieved by adjusting the positive end-expiratory pressure (PEEP) dial on the cap of the T-piece or the flow-control valve to 5–6 cmH_2O pressure. *Do not* occlude the T-piece cap or squeeze the flow-inflating bag.

If the baby cannot maintain an HR of 100 beats/min with spontaneous respirations, you need to give PPV instead of CPAP (*Note:* CPAP may increase the chance of developing a pneumothorax).

Use of orogastric tube: During CPAP or PPV with a face mask or laryngeal mask, gas enters the esophagus and stomach. Place an orogastric tube and leave it uncapped (acts as a vent for the stomach) if CPAP or PPV is needed for a longer time as gas in the stomach may interfere with ventilation.

ENDOTRACHEAL INTUBATION[3,10]

Endotracheal intubation is recommended:

- If bag-mask ventilation is ineffective or needed for a prolonged time
- Before starting CCs
- For surfactant administration, in a newborn with suspected diaphragmatic hernia, for direct tracheal suction if the trachea is obstructed by thick secretions.

Timing: Depends on the skill of the provider.

Size varies with gestational age (*2.5 mm:* Weight <1 kg/gestational age <28 weeks, *3.0 mm:* weight 1–2 kg/age 28–34 weeks, *3.5 mm:* Weight >2 kg/ age >34 weeks).

Laryngoscope blade depends on the gestation (No. 1—term babies, No. 0—preterms, and No. 00—extreme preterms).

Always check the light of the laryngoscope before attempting intubation.

After endotracheal intubation and administration of intermittent positive pressure, a prompt increase in HR is the best indicator that the tube is in the tracheobronchial tree.

If initial attempts at intubation fail or are unsuccessful in improving the HR and respiration, resume PPV with a bag and mask and then try again.

Chest Compressions[3,10,11] (Figs. 2A and B)

- *Indicated* when the HR is below 60 beats/min despite 30 seconds of effective PPV. Intubation *must* be done at this time.
- *Two techniques* used—the thumb technique (where the two thumbs are used to depress the sternum while the hands encircle the torso and fingers support the spine) or the two-finger technique (where the tips of the middle and either ring or index finger of one hand are used to compress the sternum, while the other hand supports the baby's back).

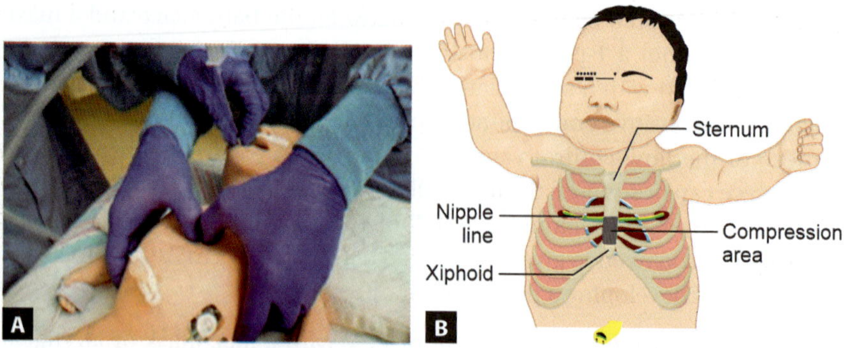

Figs. 2A and B: *Chest compressions:* (A) Landmarks for CC; (B) Two thumbs technique.

The thumb technique is preferred as one can control the depth of compression and consistent pressure is applied.

- *Site:* Lower one-third of the sternum, which lies between the xiphoid and a line drawn between the nipples.
- *Pressure:* Just enough to depress the sternum to a depth of approximately one-third the anterior-posterior diameter of the chest.

Coordination of CC with ventilation?

During CPR, CCs must always be accompanied by PPV. Both must be coordinated so that there must be one ventilation after every third compression (30 breaths and 90 compressions/min). To achieve the correct rate, use the rhythm 'One- and-Two-and-Three-and Breathe-and...."

Two people are needed, one standing at the head end to deliver PPV and one on the baby's side for CC. It is important to wait for at least 45–60 seconds of coordinated compressions and PPV before one checks the HR. The CCs are stopped if the HR rises above 60 beats/min. Continue PPV till the HR rises above 100 beats/min and there is spontaneous respiration.[3,10]

If the HR remains <60 beats/min despite 60 seconds of effective ventilation with coordinated CC, drugs are administered.

MEDICATIONS[3,10]

Rarely indicated in newborn resuscitation. However, if the HR remains <60 beats/min despite adequate ventilation with 100% oxygen and CC, administration of epinephrine and/or volume expansion, may be indicated.

Epinephrine

- *Indicated if the baby's HR remains <60 beats/min after:* At least 30 seconds of PPV that inflates the lungs as evidenced by chest movement and another 60 seconds of CC coordinated with PPV using 100% oxygen.

By now, ventilation should have been provided through a properly inserted endotracheal tube.

- *Concentration:* 1:10,000 (0.1 mg/mL).
- *Route:* Intravenous (IV) (preferred) using an umbilical venous catheter or via an intraosseous (IO) needle.
- *Dose:* 0.01–0.03 mg/kg per dose (equals 0.1–0.3 mL/kg) for IV/IO use. Follow up the dose with a 3 mL flush of normal saline.

If the *endotracheal route* is used, the dose is 0.05–0.1 mg/kg (equals 0.5–1 mL/kg), but the safety and efficacy of this practice has not been evaluated.

Volume Expander[1]

Indications

The baby may be in hypovolemic shock in cases of acute fetomaternal hemorrhage, bleeding vasa previa, extensive vaginal bleeding, placental laceration, fetal trauma, umbilical cord prolapses, a tight nuchal cord, or blood loss from the umbilical cord.

There may be a persistently low HR not responding to effective ventilation, CC, and epinephrine, and the baby may have pale skin, poor perfusion, and weak pulses.

An isotonic crystalloid solution (normal saline or ringer lactate) or blood (O negative) is recommended.

Route

The route should be intravenous or IO.

Dose: 10 mL/kg, over 5–10 minutes (may be repeated).

POSTRESUSCITATION CARE

Babies who require resuscitation are at risk for deterioration. Hence, they should be kept in a place where close monitoring and care are provided.

CONCLUSION

The NRP guidelines have been published taking into account the availability of the best possible services and the latest equipment found in developing countries. In a country like ours, this may not be always possible. The Indian Academy of Pediatrics-National Neonatology Forum (IAP-NNF) National Task Force 2006 recommends starting PPV in cases of meconium even at a slight fall in HR rather than waiting for a fall below 60 beats/min. Studies showing room air resuscitation being as effective as O_2 is an advantage. Also, the use of IO infusions, an art learned by paramedics rather than IV access works in the field. Making a few modifications as per the country's status can help improve their neonatal mortality rates.

REFERENCES

1. American Heart Association and American Academy of Paediatrics. In: Weiner GM, Zaichkin J (Eds). Textbook of Neonatal Resuscitation, 8th edition. New Delhi: CBS Publications; 2021.
2. National Health Mission, Ministry of Health and Family Welfare, Government Of India. (2020). Navjaat Shishu Suraksha Kaaryakram. [online] Available from https://nhm.gov.in/images/pdf/programmes/child health/guidelines/NSSK/NSSK-Resource-Manual.pdf [Last accessed August, 2024].
3. Shah NK, Mathur NB, et al. Neonatal resuscitation. IAP-NNF guidelines 2006 on level II neonatal care. 2006;3-13.
4. In: Kattwinkel J, McGowan JE, Zaichkin J (Eds). Overview and principles of resuscitation. Textbook of neonatal resuscitation, 6th edition. New Delhi: Jaypee Brothers Medical Publishers; 2012; pp. 1-36.
5. American Academy of Pediatrics, American College of Obstetricians and Gynecologists. In: Gilstrap LC, Oh W (Eds). Guidelines for Perinatal Care, 5th edition. Elk Grove Village, III: American Academy of Pediatrics; 2002. p. 187.
6. Morley CJ, Davis PG, Doyle LW, Brion LP, Hascoet JM, Carlin JB. Nasal CPAP or intubation at birth for very preterm infants. N Engl J Med. 2008;358(7):700-8.
7. Finer NN, Rich W, Craft A, Henderson C. Comparison of methods bag and mask ventilation for neonatal resuscitation. Resuscitation. 2001;49:299-305.
8. Benett S, Finer NN, Rich W, Vaucher Y. A comparison of three neonatal resuscitation devices. Resuscitation. 2005;67(1):113-8.
9. Rabi Y, Rabi D, Yee W. Room air resuscitation of the depressed newborn: a systematic review and meta-analysis. Resuscitation. 2007;72(3):353-63.
10. Kattwinkel J, Perlman JM, Aziz K, Colby C, Fairchild K, Gallagher J, et al. Part 15: neonatal resuscitation: 2010 American Heart Association Guidelines for Cardiopulmonary Resuscitation and Emergency Cardiovascular Care. Circulation. 2010;122(18 Suppl 3):S909-19.
11. Orlowski JP. Optimum position for external cardiac compression in infants and young children. Ann Emerg Med. 1986;15(6):667-73.

CHAPTER 2

Current Practice of Cesarean Section

Suchitra Pandit, Deepali Prakash Kale, Aditya Rajiv Nimbkar

INTRODUCTION

Cesarean section (CS) is a method of delivering the fetus via the abdominal route. It is an essential component of good quality intrapartum care, yet it carries inherent risks for women and newborns.

The first CS took place in 1020 AD, and surgeries have evolved since then.[1]

The cesarean section rates (CSR) have increased at an alarming rate globally as well as in India, thereby posing a burden on overstretched health systems.

Improved operative techniques, better suture materials, expert anesthesia, potent antibiotics, availability of blood transfusion facilities, and better neonatal care contribute to quicker recovery periods, which have helped in improved outcomes of CS. This has resulted in a steady and definite rise in the incidence of CS.

Despite the high numbers of CS performed globally, modifications in the techniques and materials used have been adapted, but the essence of this surgery has been preserved. There is an increase in maternal and perinatal morbidity and mortality compared to an uncomplicated vaginal delivery (VD). Possible side effects for the mother such as fever, infection or bleeding, and complications in subsequent pregnancies. Increased susceptibility to allergies, atopic and asthmatic conditions, and reduced gut microbiome diversity, including changes in the immune system in infants.[2,3] The risk of maternal death is also increased when CS is performed without medical advice.[4]

Many efforts are being made to reduce CSR, yet experts in the field do not expect the rate to drop for at least another decade or two.[5]

THE CHANGING TRENDS IN CESAREAN SECTION: THE HISTORICAL TIMELINE

The National Family Health Survey (NFHS) released data in 2021 after surveying a sample of 230,870 women in India between 2019 and 2021, which revealed that CSR has increased from 3% in 1992–1993 to 21.5% in 2019–2021.[6,7]

National Family Health Survey[7] generates national population-based data depending on the health indicators, especially on maternal and child health which is equivalent to the Health Survey of India.

TABLE 1: NFHS[4,5] births delivered by cesarean section (%).[7]

Urban	*Rural*	*Total (2015–2016)*	*Total (2020–2021)*
32.3	17.6	17.2	21.5

According to NFHS 4 and NFHS 5,[7] there is a rise in CSR with changing patterns of indications as well as changes in the proportion of public and private sectors **(Table 1)**. The accepted international surgery rate is 10–15% [World Health Organization (WHO)].[8]

DIFFERENCE BETWEEN PRIVATE AND PUBLIC SECTOR CESAREAN SECTION RATES

There is a disparity in the rates between various socioeconomic groups, like 47.4% in private institutions versus 14.3% in public hospitals, 32.3% in urban settings versus 17.6% in rural settings.[7]

The odds of performing CS were 40% higher in private hospitals than in public hospitals after adjusting for other known confounding risk factors.

These statistics reveal that few hospitals have a much lower threshold for indications for CS and a certain rise in possibly unindicated surgeries.

An Evolutionary Perspective

From an evolutionary perspective, human birth is considered an event in which the parturient is accompanied by social support which will reduce anxiety and possibly curtail unnecessary operative interventions during labor.[9,10]

IMPLICATIONS OF RISING CESAREAN SECTION RATE

Cesarean sections have been offered given maternal and fetal health safety in the following cases:

- *Maternal indications* such as placenta previa, antepartum hemorrhage, anticipated traumatic delivery, and morbid adhesions of the placenta.
- *Fetal indications* such as malpresentations, fetal distress, cord accidents in early labor, large fetus (>4 kg in a diabetic mother and >5 kg in a nondiabetic mother)
- *Current indications* for performing CS include the use of electronic fetal monitoring, previous CR, older women getting pregnant and having medical conditions such as gestational diabetes and pregnancy-induced hypertension, a rising rate of multiple pregnancies due to assisted techniques of reproduction (ART) use of lateral metroplasty previous bad obstetric history or ART pregnancies, malpresentations such as breech and transverse lie, failure to progress and failure of induction.

With better neonatal intensive care units, if emergency delivery in complicated preterm pregnancies is required CS is used.

So, summarizing the causes for a high CSR:

- Increased perceived fetal safety of CS over VD
- Cesarean delivery on maternal request (CDMR) due to fear of the pain associated with VD and other social factors
- Desire to deliver on an auspicious day and time
- Increased levels of education and ability of families to afford CS
- Obstetricians' fear of medicolegal implications about poor fetal outcomes due to VD

Methods to Address Rising Rates of Cesarean Section

Various methods can be adopted to address these rising rates of CS:

- State Health Policy should plan to reduce cesarean births by increasing knowledge and awareness about maternal health among women and communities through community health workers and primary care providers. Recommending lifestyle changes, having a balanced diet, and encouraging physical activities especially in urban areas to maintain a healthy weight gain in pregnancy especially if body mass index (BMI) is >30.
- The WHO statement proposes the use of Robson's classification as the global standard for assessing, monitoring, and comparing cesarean rates, over time within healthcare facilities and between facilities in a more action-oriented and meaningful manner.

CLINICAL INTERVENTIONS

- Offering external cephalic versions for breech presentation
- Vaginal birth after cesarean section (VBAC)
- Trial of labor after CS in selected cases after counseling patients
- Training audits and regular skill upgrading in continuous cardiotocography (CTG) interpretation
- Use of assisted VD with the help of forceps or vacuum and training of the resident doctors for these techniques
- Use of the WHO—next generation partograph[10] **(Fig. 1)**

Nonclinical Interventions

The WHO labor care guide—issued by the WHO:[10]

- Use of doulas (labor assistants) and constant caring companion
- Oral hydration
- Mobility during the first stage
- Birth position of choice
- Pain management
- Respectful maternal care
- Informed decision making

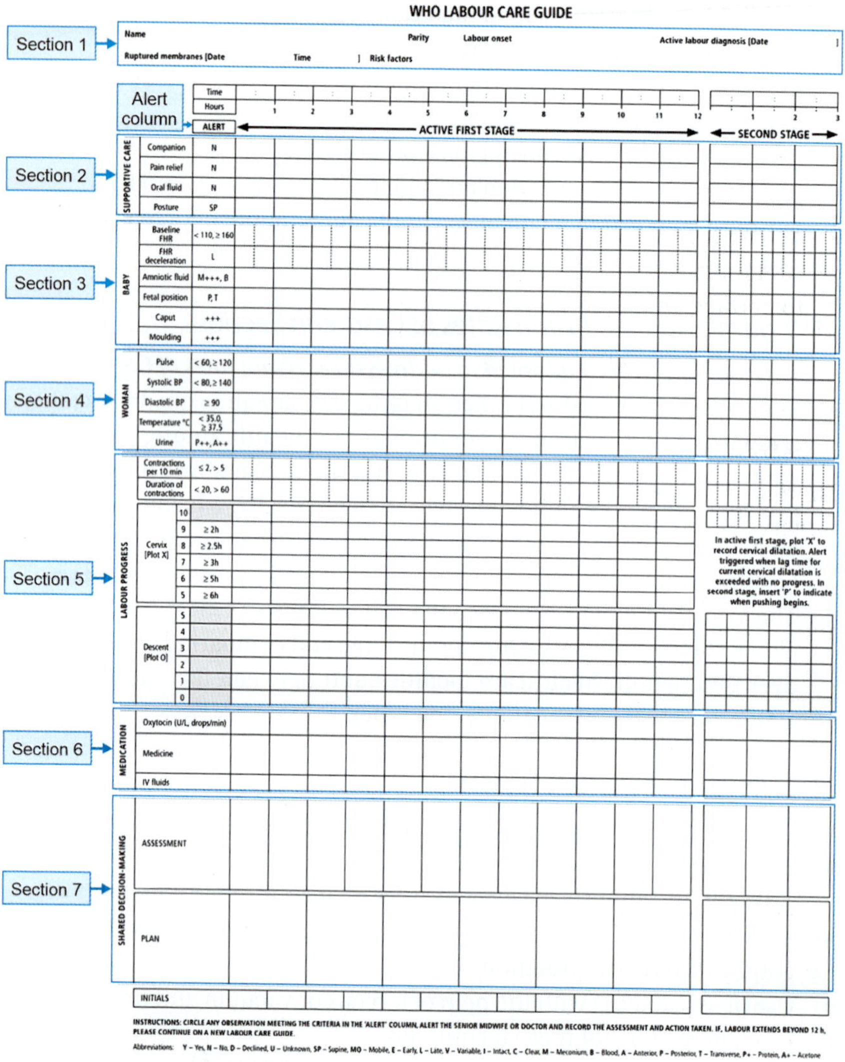

Fig. 1: World Health Organization (WHO) next-generation partograph.[10]

Nonclinical interventions are presumably useful in reducing CSR:

- Providing adequate knowledge to the women and their families and developing better communication with them
- The best consensus among labor care guide (LCG) is the midwifery collaboration in conjunction with more births, maternal and fetal safety quality of birth for mothers and reduced costs.

Caregivers support the woman's role in the reduction of cesarean birth by providing clarity on risks and benefits to enable women to make the best choices regarding their birth.

SPECIAL KEY FEATURES OF WHO NEXT GENERATION PARTOGRAPH

- Active labor is to be assessed from a cervical dilatation of 5 cm and each of the subsequent centimeters of dilatation will be allotted its period for progression before the decision for nonprogress of labor for CS is made.
- The additional provision of an accompanying person with the laboring woman to ease the process and encourage the use of obstetric analgesia to reduce the pain and psychological discomfort for the pregnant women.

ENHANCED RECOVERY PROGRAMS AFTER SURGERY[11] (FIG. 2)

There is also an increased acceptance of the enhanced recovery after surgery (ERAS) protocols in recent times. It intends to reduce postoperative hospital stays, and rates of perioperative complications and improve patient satisfaction. There are three segments: (1) Preoperative, (2) intraoperative, and (3) postoperative periods.[11]

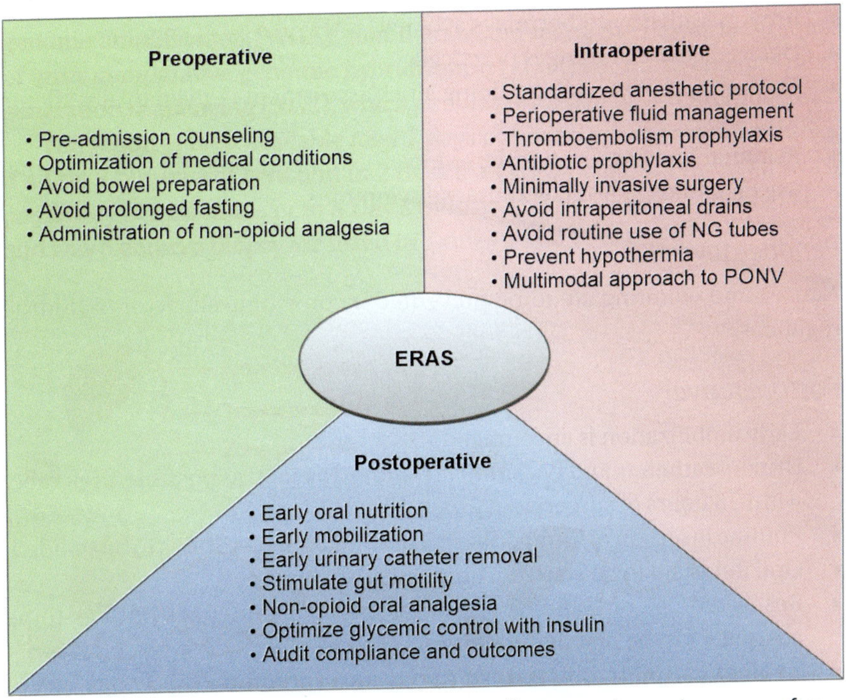

Fig. 2: Enhanced recovery program after surgery.[11] (ERAS: enhanced recovery after surgery; NG: nasogastric; PONV: postoperative nausea and vomiting)

Preoperative Segment

- Patient education and counseling regarding the CS, indication, and its alternatives are explained.
- A patient can have solid food items till 2 hours before surgery and clear, complex-carbohydrate-rich oral fluids to reduce the postoperative thirst till 2 hours of surgery. This reduces the need for prolonged starvation, which predisposes to electrolyte imbalance.
- Preoperative optimization of the patient's fitness and hemoglobin and other necessary investigations. Bathing in the night before surgery is advised.
- Clipping is recommended instead of shaving off the hair, in the operative field.
- Counseling for breastfeeding

Intraoperative Segment

- Intravenous (IV) antibiotics are given an hour before the skin incision, and a repeat dose is given intraoperatively if blood loss exceeds 1,500 mL or operative time exceeds 3 hours.
- Surgical parts are cleaned using chlorhexidine, preferably over povidone iodine to reduce the risk of infection at the surgery site, and shorten hospital stay and readmissions.
- Intraoperative hypothermia is avoided.
- Delayed cord clamping is practiced.
- Thromboprophylaxis after doing a risk assessment is given to all patients who had a CS.
- Regional anesthesia is preferred over general anesthesia with minimal use of opioids to avoid withdrawal symptoms.

Perioperative

Nausea and vomiting are to be prevented by providing single or multidrug regimens.

Postoperative

- Early mobilization is encouraged.
- Urinary catheters and IV cannulae removed as soon as possible, preferably within 6 hours of surgery.
- Routine insertion of intraperitoneal or subcutaneous drains to be avoided.
- Oral fluids are to be started within one hour of surgery.
- Restricted use of IV fluids once oral intake commences but has to be adequate for the first day of surgery.
- Analgesics, preferably nonsteroidal anti-inflammatory drugs are to be given.
- Thus, ERAS helps to ensure a swift recovery period for a patient with CS.

Advances Regarding Techniques of Cesarean Section

The number of emergency CSs performed in the second stage is increasing The risk of complications for the mother and the baby is substantially higher due to manipulations needed for delivering the fetus than elective CS or CS done earlier. Currently, there is no national consensus on which techniques to use for the delivery of an impacted fetal head at CS.

Novel Innovation for Baby Delivery (MIDAS Trial)[12]

A fetal pillow, a contemporary cephalic elevation device, is used in the United Kingdom for CS in case of full dilatation to push up the deeply impacted head to reduce fetal and maternal morbidity and mortality **(Fig. 3)**.

This device is placed in the vagina before a CS, and inflated with normal saline so it elevates the head, which was otherwise deeply impacted in the pelvis.

The trial comparing the new device with the method of manually pushing the impacted fetal head through the vagina showed a reduction in fetal and maternal morbidity and operating times.

Patwardhan's technique: Resident Doctors globally must be trained in Patwardhan's surgical technique (from India) of delivery of shoulders when there is a deeply impacted head. Training can be given in skill labs with dummies and later assisting experienced clinicians and finally doing it under expert supervision.

CORONIS Trial[13]

CORONIS trial was a large randomized trial of CS procedures aimed to assess whether any surgical techniques were associated with improved outcomes for women and babies. Each site was assigned to three of the five intervention pairs: (1) Blunt versus sharp abdominal entry; (2) Exteriorization of the uterus

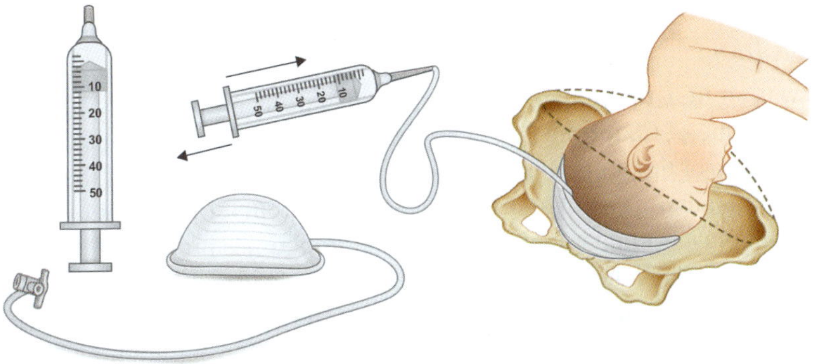

Fig. 3: Fetal pillow (fetal disimpacting system).[12]

for repair versus intra-abdominal repair; (3) Single-layer versus double-layer closure of the uterus; (4) Closure versus nonclosure of the peritoneum; and (5) Chromic catgut versus Polyglactin-910 for uterine repair. Pregnant women undergoing their first or second CS through a planned transverse abdominal incision were eligible.

There were no significant differences in outcome for any pair of interventions. Cases using Polyglactin 910 fared better than those where chromic catgut was used for uterine incision repair.

CORONIS findings suggest that any of these surgical techniques is acceptable but long-term follow-up is needed to assess whether the absence of evidence of short-term effects will translate into an absence of long-term effects.

DECIDE (Decision for Cesarean Delivery) Trial[14]

This was a cluster randomized controlled trial (RCT) of a multifaceted intervention at 22 referral hospitals in Burkina Faso (West Africa—a low-income country). This is the first attempt to validate the benefits of using evidence-based assessment methods to improve CS and was targeted at healthcare professionals. It included availability and training on evidence-based algorithms for cesarean decision-making, audits of cesarean indications with timely feedback to healthcare professionals, and SMS reminders, resulting in a significant reduction in unnecessary CSs and improved the quality of decision-making for it.

The DECIDE intervention improved doctors' performance due to improvement in decision-making quality scores working with different skills.

It was also associated with a significant decrease in the relative contributions of Robson groups 1 and 3 (women with a single cephalic pregnancy at term in spontaneous labor without a previous CS) to the overall CSR. The intervention did not significantly affect the rates of maternal or intrapartum neonatal mortality among cesarean births.

CESAR Trial[15]

This was an RCT to evaluate two alternative approaches to three aspects of the technique of CS for the risk of adverse outcomes: Single-versus double-layer closure of the uterine incision; closure versus nonclosure of the pelvic peritoneum; liberal versus restricted use of a subrectus sheath drain.

Results suggest that nonclosure of the peritoneum is preferable.

The potential effects of these different surgical techniques on long-term outcomes including the functional integrity of the uterine scar during subsequent pregnancies, are now becoming important for guiding clinical practice.

CESAREAN SECTION AND LONG-TERM EFFECTS

Maternal

Having a CS increases the risk of complications in later pregnancy and in other surgeries. The more the CSs, the higher the risks of uterine rupture, stillbirth placenta previa and morbid placental adhesions, ectopic pregnancy, preterm birth, post-traumatic stress disorder, and postpartum depression. These risks increase in a dose-response manner.

Short-term risks of CS include altered immune development, an increased likelihood of allergy, asthma, and reduced intestinal gut microbiome diversity. Whether they persist in later life for long is not yet studied.

Fetal

- Many studies have shown that children born by CS have a higher risk of obesity than those born vaginally.
- Childhood obesity assesses the difference in plasma biomarker levels of metabolic health and inflammation in children born by CS compared to vaginal birth in middle childhood and early childhood.[16]

CESAREAN DELIVERY AT THE MOTHER'S REQUEST[17,18]

A primary elective cesarean delivery is performed at term in a singleton pregnancy without any obstetric and/or medical reasons.

The perception of CS as the painless and safest way to give birth, and the movement of giving voice and respecting the autonomy of pregnant women contribute to the increased rates of CDMR. This cannot simply be labeled as "not medically necessary."

Factors influencing CDMR are multifactorial:

- Anxiety and fear of the labor pain and vaginal birth
- Previous poor labor experience
- Concerns about fetal injury or stillbirth from previous vaginal birth
- Concerns about trauma to the pelvic floor; and laxity in later life
- Convenience of scheduled and planned birth
- Shorter delivery time without labor pain.
- Lack of knowledge about the risks and benefits of a CS

The obstetrician's job is to provide the patient with adequate information and support her in her decision. This should be based on the principle of premium non-nocere (not harm) and should advise against dangerous procedures. Surgeons have the right to refuse unnecessary surgery.[19,20]

The conflict between the principle of nonmaleficence and the patient's autonomy[19] needs to be taken into consideration during patient counseling or can lead to legal problems.

Obstetric practice appears to be influenced by the fear of being sued, and procedures are being designed to reduce discomfort.[18-20] It is often evident that in situations of doubt, fear, and conflict, doctors prefer to minimize the risk of litigation.[21]

As a result, the incidence of VBAC, operative deliveries, and breech birth has decreased and more CS is performed to reduce the risk of the perceived difficult labor processes. This "defensive attitude is also taken when some doctors wish to avoid difficult or controversial patients.[22]

TOKOPHOBIA

There is a severe fear of childbirth, around 14% which affects the participation of the parturient in the process of labor.[23] It may be correlated with a previous traumatic birth or any stress factor like a childhood trauma (emotional, psychological, or sexual abuse) which be related to anxiety and depression. This fear is also thought to originate from the fear of uncertainty and the unknown.[24,25]

- When a woman requests a cesarean delivery, the reasons for her request must be identified, discussed, and documented.
- All guidelines recommend that healthcare professionals must do proper counseling of women and their families requesting CDMR. Understanding the reasons, and providing evidence-based information on the risks and benefits of elective CS compared with the risks and benefits of VD. Respecting the patient's autonomy and keeping ethical principles in mind is important.
- The mode of birth should be discussed during early pregnancy to identify the prospective risk group of women who may need more counseling and support around childbirth.
- Encouraging prenatal classes for couples, teaching analgesia, relaxation exercises, birth preparation, and mental health education to help them decide about delivery.
- Training of health professionals from experienced doctors especially in the use of clinical guidelines in conjunction with audits and feedback on CS practice.

INTERVENTIONS TARGETING HEALTHCARE ORGANIZATIONS OR FACILITIES[26,27]

Interventions Targeted at Women

- Childbirth training programs—which provide information about fear and pain during childbirth, effective drugs, and nonpharmacological methods for pain relief.

- *Programs of nurse-led applied relaxation techniques* to reduce stress and anxiety during pregnancy.
- *Psychoreduction* by a therapist and a midwife to reduce fear of pain and anxiety related to childbirth.
- *Psychological couple-based prevention program* to help in conflict management and building positive attitudes.

Interventions Targeted at Healthcare Professionals

Implementation of evidence-based clinical practice guidelines, and mandatory second opinions for CS indications from senior clinicians is recommended to reduce cesarean births in settings with adequate resources.

Interventions Targeted at Health Organizations, Facilities, or Systems

The WHO recommends the midwife-obstetrician partnership model of care receiving 24-hour support from obstetricians.

- Audits and feedback about upgrading the skills and competencies in CTG interpretation to avoid false positive CTG.
- Training of resident doctors for instrumental VD, in skill laboratories, later, assisting and later performing under observation by the consultant which will reduce the second stage CS.

LEGAL PERSPECTIVE

The fear of litigation has led the clinicians to opt for defensive practices which are performed more likely as the actions taken to reduce the likelihood of being sued rather than to help the patient.[28,29] So following evidence-based guidelines and improving communication skills for a better doctor-patient relationship will help to reduce this fear.

SUMMARY

- The use of CS has been steadily increasing worldwide and will continue to do so, where both, unmet need and overuse are expected to coexist which drains resources and adds to the avoidable morbidity and mortality.
- To reach sustainable development goals within the next decade, addressing the CS issue is a global priority, generating awareness and advocating for appropriate, evidence-based, and respectful care during pregnancy and childbirth.
- WHO urges that every attempt should be made to provide CS only to women in need. It is essential to counsel and provide adequate information to the woman to help her make an informed choice, ensure supportive care to the woman, and finally respect her autonomy.

- Use of evidence-based guidelines and improving communication skills for a better doctor-patient relationship will help to reduce this fear of litigations.
- Adopting nonclinical and clinical strategies such as support groups and audits, training, and increase uptake of instrumental vaginal deliveries to reduce CSR.

REFERENCES

1. Berghella V, Baxter JK, Chauhan SP. Evidence-based surgery for cesarean delivery. Am J Obstet Gynecol. 2005;193(5):1607-17.
2. Brach DW, Silver RM. Managing the primary cesarean delivery rate. Clin Obstet Gynecol. 2012;55(4):946-60.
3. Sandall J, Tribe RM, Avery L, Mola G, Visser GHA, Homer CSE, et al. Short-term and long-term effects of caesarean section on the health of women and children. Lancet. 2018;392(10155):1349-57.
4. Souza JP, Gülmezoglu A, Lumbiganon P, Laopaiboon M, Carroli G, Fawole B, et al. Caesarean section without medical indications is associated with an increased risk of adverse short-term maternal outcomes: the 2004-2008 WHO Global Survey on Maternal and Perinatal Health. BMC Med. 2010;8:71.
5. Clapp MA, Barth WH. The future of cesarean delivery rates in the United States. Clin Obstet Gynecol. 2017;60(4):829-39.
6. Simmons E, Lane K, Rao SR, Kurhe K, Patel A, Hibberd PL. Trends in cesarean section rates in private and public facilities in rural eastern Maharashtra, India from 2010–2017. PLoS One. 2021;16(8):e0256096.
7. IIPS/India and ICF. (2017). National Family Health Survey NFHS-4, 2015-16. [Online] Available from https://dhsprogram.com/pubs/pdf/FR339/FR339.pdf [Last accessed August, 2024].
8. World Health Organization (WHO). WHO statement on caesarean section rates. Geneva: World Health Organization; 2015. [Online] Available from: https://apps.who.int/iris/bitstream/handle/10665/161442/WHO_RHR_15.02_eng.pdf?sequence=1 [Last accessed August, 2024].
9. Rosenberg KR, Trevathan WR. Evolutionary perspectives on cesarean section: evolution, medicine, and public health. 2018;2018(1):67-81.
10. Vogel JP, Pingray V, Althabe F, Gibbons L, Berrueta M, Pujar Y, et al. Implementing the WHO Labour Care Guide to reduce the use of caesarean section in four hospitals in India: protocol and statistical analysis plan for a pragmatic, stepped-wedge, cluster-randomized pilot trial. Reprod Health. 2023;20(1):18.
11. He L, Lu L, Su S, Lin Q, Sheng C. Top 100 most-cited articles on enhanced recovery after surgery: a bibliometric analysis and visualized study. Front Surg. 2022;9:845946.
12. Walker KF, Mitchell EJ, Ayers S, Jones NW, Ogollah R, Wakefield N, et al. Feasibility of a RCT of techniques for managing an impacted fetal head during emergency caesarean section: the MIDAS scoping study. Health Technol Assess. 2023;27(6):1-87.
13. Abalos E, Addo V, Brocklehurst P, El Sheikh M, Farrell B, Gray S, et al. Caesarean section surgical techniques (CORONIS): a fractional, factorial, unmasked, randomised controlled trial. Lancet. 2013;382(9888):234-48.

14. Kaboré C, Ridde V, Chaillet N, Yaya Bocoum F, Betrán AP, Dumont A. DECIDE: a cluster-randomized controlled trial to reduce unnecessary caesarean deliveries in Burkina Faso. BMC Med. 2019;17(1):87.
15. The CAESAR Study Collaborative Group. Caesarean section surgical techniques: a randomised factorial trial (CAESAR). BJOG. 2010;117(11):1366-76.
16. Mínguez-Alarcón L, Rifas-Shiman SL, Mitchell C, Sordillo J, Aris IM, Hivert MF, et al. Cesarean delivery and metabolic health and inflammation biomarkers during mid-childhood and early adolescence. Pediatr Res. 2022;91(3):672-80.
17. American College of Obstetricians and Gynecologists ACOG Committee Opinion No. 394, December 2007. Cesarean delivery on maternal request. Obstet Gynecol. 2007;110(6):1501.
18. Sorrentino F, Greco F, Palieri T, Vasciaveo L, Stabile G, Carlucci S, et al. Caesarean Section on Maternal Request-Ethical and Juridic Issues: a narrative review. Medicina (Kaunas). 2022;58(9):1255.
19. Romanis EC. Why the elective caesarean lottery is ethically impermissible? Health Care Anal. 2019;27(4):249-68.
20. Indraccolo U, Scutiero G, Matteo M, Indraccolo SR, Greco P. Cesarean section on maternal request: should it be formally prohibited in Italy? Ann Ist Super Sanita. 2015;51(2):162-6.
21. Minkoff H. Fear of litigation and cesarean section rates. Semin Perinatol. 2012;36(5):390-94.
22. Rybak EA. Hippocratic ideal, Faustian bargain and Damocles' sword: Erosion of patient autonomy in obstetrics. J Perinatol. 2009;29(11):721-5.
23. O'Connell MA, Leahy-Warren P, Khashan AS, Kenny LC, O'Neill SM. Worldwide prevalence of tocophobia in pregnant women: systematic review and meta-analysis. Acta Obstet Gynecol Scand. 2017;96(8):907-20.
24. Söderquist J, Wijma B, Thorbert G, Wijma K. Risk factors in pregnancy for post-traumatic stress and depression after childbirth. Int J Obstet Gynaecol. 2009;116(5):672-80.
25. Molgora S, Fenaroli V, Prino LE, Rollè L, Sechi C, Trovato A, et al. Fear of childbirth in primiparous Italian pregnant women: the role of anxiety, depression, and couple adjustment. Women Birth. 2018;31(12):117-23.
26. Opiyo N, Kingdon C, Oladapo OT, Souza JP, Vogel JP, Bonet M, et al. Non-clinical interventions to reduce unnecessary caesarean sections: WHO recommendations. Bull World Health Organ. 2020;98(1):66-8.
27. Chen I, Opiyo N, Tavender E, Mortazhejri S, Rader T, Petkovic J, et al. Non-clinical interventions for reducing unnecessary caesarean section. Cochrane Database Syst Rev. 2018;9(9):CD005528.
28. Ionescu CA, Dimitriu M, Poenaru E, Bănacu M, Furău GO, Navolan D, et al. Defensive caesarean section: a reality and a recommended health care improvement for Romanian obstetrics. J Eval Clin Pract. 2019;25(1):111-6.
29. Asher E, Dvir S, Seidman DS, Greenberg-Dotan S, Kedem A, Sheizaf B, et al. Defensive medicine among obstetricians and gynecologists in tertiary hospitals. PLoS ONE. 2013;8(3):e57108.

CHAPTER 3

Pregnancy after ART

Charmila Ayyavoo

INTRODUCTION

The incidence of conceptions using assisted reproductive technology (ART) has increased tremendously over the years. It has risen from 230,000 in the year 2003 to 439,000 in the year 2014.[1,2]

Assisted conceptions are known to be associated with an increased risk of maternal and fetal complications. Obstetricians involved in the care of ART pregnancies must have a clear understanding of the risks involved and the ideal way of monitoring and managing such pregnancies. The complications in a pregnancy following ART usually occur in multiple pregnancies. However, singleton ART pregnancies are also associated with increasing morbidity in the mother and the baby.[3]

The causes for the increased maternal and fetal morbidity may be due to the procedures done during ART, the medications, the altered uterine endocrine environment during implantation, or the manipulations of the gametes and the embryos. There may be a combination of factors. There is also no clarity on whether this is a consequence of the procedures involved in ART or due to the innate characteristics of the patients who undertake them.[4]

The continuity of care in the antenatal period of an ART pregnancy is very important. A system of clear referral paths should be established so that pregnant women who require additional care are managed and treated by the appropriate specialist teams when problems are identified.

COMPLICATIONS IN ART PREGNANCIES

The complications may be maternal as well as fetal. Medical disorders in pregnancy and obstetric complications are common in ART pregnancies.

There is a higher incidence of hypertensive disorders in pregnancy (HDP), hyperglycemia in pregnancy (HIP), thyroid disorders, and thromboembolic episodes. The risk factors contributing to maternal complications are pregnancies at older ages, association of a higher body mass index (BMI), polycystic ovarian disease, multiple pregnancies, and pregnancies that are created from oocyte, sperm, or embryo donation.

Hypertensive Disorders in Pregnancy and ART

The use of ART treatment is associated with a 1.71-fold increase in preeclampsia (PE).[5] It can happen in ART pregnancies per se even with no other risk factor. HDP is seen more in donor oocyte programs with a higher incidence in frozen cycles.

The Gestosis score used for the screening for HDP gives a score of one for pregnancies conceived through ART. The score is three if the pregnancies are through ovum donation or surrogacy. A score of 3 according to the Federation of Obstetric and Gynaecological Societies of India (FOGSI), Indian College of Obstetricians and Gynaecologists (ICOG), and good clinical practice recommendations (GCPR) on HDP indicates a high risk for developing HDP in that pregnancy.[6]

Abnormal placentation in ART pregnancies may be a reason for the development of hypertension. In some ART procedures, the blood flow is compromised and diminished, which is then followed by obstetric complications. Placental insufficiency can occur because of the altered hormonal environment in the endometrium. It has been argued that ART may have epigenetic effects.

Donor Gametes and Hypertension in Pregnancy

Pregnancies conceived through donor oocytes show an increased risk for preeclampsia. There is a 25% incidence of preeclampsia in donor gamete pregnancies. The placenta may not be the villain in each case of preeclampsia. The role of maternal immune reaction against alien antigens of the fetus may play a role in the high incidence of HDP in donor gestations.[7]

Frozen Cycles and HDP

Artificial frozen embryo transfer (FET) cycles have an increased preeclampsia risk in comparison with natural and stimulated cycles. It has been proposed that the absence of the corpus luteum in artificial cycles may contribute to the observed increased risk of preeclampsia. The corpus luteum secretes vasoactive hormones, such as relaxin, which are not replaced in artificial cycles, thereby compromising maternal cardiovascular adaptations to pregnancy, resulting in an increased risk of preeclampsia.[8]

Recurrent pregnancy losses and miscarriages are high in ART conceptions. It is also associated with an increased risk of preeclampsia in these pregnancies. Pregnancies from ART are associated with preeclampsia through oxidative stress. In addition, ART has several types of reproductive dysfunction with the same strength as miscarriages. Recurrent spontaneous miscarriages, along with infertility treatments, increase the risk of preeclampsia in comparison to those without treatment. Women who conceive multiple gestations through assisted reproductive technologies have a 2.1-fold higher risk of preeclampsia than those who conceive spontaneously. For women receiving in vitro fertilization (IVF)/intracytoplasmic sperm injection (ICSI), lower estradiol hormone levels on the day of human chorionic gonadotropin (hCG) administration and higher pregnancy weight gain are related to subsequent preeclampsia.[9]

There is also an association of adenomyosis with ART and HDP. Women with adenomyosis and who have undergone ICSI show signs of uteroplacental malperfusion during the first trimester and possibly have an increased risk of preeclampsia and composite adverse perinatal outcomes.[10]

Assisted reproductive technology is an independent risk factor for developing gestational diabetes mellitus (GDM). The risk for GDM increases more in overweight and obese women who have undergone ART.[11]

VENOUS THROMBOEMBOLISM

The American College of Clinical Pharmacy-Clinical Practice Guidelines (ACCP-CPG) found that while ART may be a risk factor, the incidence of thrombosis in ART patients was low. However, the risk of thrombosis was found to be higher in women with ovarian hyperstimulation syndrome (OHSS). The ACCP-CPG recommends against routine thromboprophylaxis for women undergoing ART. For those who develop severe OHSS, thromboprophylaxis for 3-months postresolution of the condition is suggested.[12]

OBSTETRIC COMPLICATIONS

Complications in early pregnancy are OHSS, miscarriages, and ectopic pregnancy. The late complications are preterm labor, stillbirth, placental complications, and increased cesarean delivery rates.[3] Fetal complications in ART pregnancies can be in the form of genetic and chromosomal disorders, structural abnormalities, growth restriction, stillbirth, and preterm labor.

MANAGEMENT OF PREGNANCIES AFTER ART

Pregnancies after ART need to be managed by specialists well-versed in high-risk obstetrics.[12] If there is a multiple pregnancy, options for fetal reduction are discussed with the couple.[13]

LUTEAL PHASE SUPPORT

The practice of luteal phase support (LPS) is established beyond doubt in patients who have undergone ART. Whatever support is administered at the point of embryo transfer should be continued till confirmation of cardiac activity on ultrasound. This includes progesterone and estrogen for oocyte recipients, embryo recipients, and frozen-thawed embryo transfer cycles. LPS is continued until 10 weeks of gestation.

MATERNAL SURVEILLANCE IN ART CONCEPTIONS

There is a higher risk of preeclampsia and preterm labor in ART pregnancies. The mother is screened for both, and preventive strategies are adopted.[14]

The confirmation of the gestational age is very important in pregnancies after ART. 2 weeks after an embryo transfer, a quantitative serum beta-hCG (β-hCG) is done, and if it suggests implantation, a transvaginal ultrasound is done to confirm the site of gestation. This is done as soon as possible as ectopic pregnancies are known to occur. In ART conceptions, heterotopic pregnancies are also common after ART. An early ultrasound will also confirm viability and chorionicity. Very high levels of β-hCG are suggestive of multiple gestations and therefore should raise the level of suspicion for all future scans.

There may be a higher risk of psychological issues in couples who have conceived by ART. The couple should be referred for psychosocial care when they experience distress regarding the pregnancy.[15]

FETAL SURVEILLANCE

Genetic and chromosomal disorders and structural abnormalities are relatively more common in ART pregnancies. A combined first-trimester screening is advisable. Nuchal translucency (NT) sonography is performed by a sonographer experienced in this technique. An assay of pregnancy-associated plasma protein A (PAPP-A) and free beta-hCG (fβ-hCG) is done. There is a higher risk of congenital malformations in ART pregnancies which include genital tract malformations, cardiac septal defects, atresia of the esophagus, and anorectal atresia in comparison to spontaneous conceptions.[16] There is also an increased risk of aneuploidy in ART pregnancies; hence, prenatal screening is advisable in all ART pregnancies according to the Society of Obstetricians and Gynaecologists of Canada (SOGC) guideline. As the risk of chromosomal abnormality is high, invasive testing can be offered without prior noninvasive screening or based on a noninvasive screening result above the risk cut-off.[14]

The ACOG guideline suggests that ultrasonographic surveillance for structural abnormalities and fetal echocardiography should be offered in all ART pregnancies, although the incremental yield is unclear. A detailed sonographic fetal anatomic survey is performed at 18–20 weeks' gestation.[17]

No additional surveillance is recommended other than a routine anomaly ultrasound scan undertaken at 18–20 + 6 weeks of gestation. Growth scans need to be done at 28 and 34 weeks of gestation. When structural problems are encountered, the possibility of subtle chromosomal rearrangements should be considered.

The miscarriage rate among pregnancies following ART is estimated to be approximately 15–20% and, like spontaneous conceptions, increases with increasing age.

The specific cause of subfertility may also affect the miscarriage rate. Congenital uterine anomalies, fibroids, and endocrine disorders are associated with higher rates of miscarriage than those without.

FETAL GROWTH RESTRICTION

Assisted reproductive technology is a minor risk factor for fetal growth restriction (FGR) and in the absence of any other risk factors, increased surveillance is not currently recommended. Maternal age ≥35 years, nulliparity, and a BMI of between 25 and 29.9 kg/m^2 are minor risk factors for fetal growth restriction.[12]

In the presence of three or more minor risk factors, a uterine artery Doppler at 20–24 weeks of gestation and an assessment of fetal size and umbilical artery Doppler in the third trimester are done.

Maternal age ≥40 years is a major risk factor and serial assessment of fetal size and umbilical artery Doppler is recommended from 26–28 weeks of gestation in these women, irrespective of how they conceived.

Pregnancies conceived using ART are associated with a significantly higher risk of placental anomalies, including placenta previa, morbidly adherent placenta, and placental abruption, compared with spontaneously conceived pregnancies.

This increase in risk is believed to be a direct effect of the ART process itself, rather than a consequence of an underlying maternal structural complication, such as Asherman's syndrome. Transfer of a cryopreserved embryo is less likely to be complicated by placenta previa.

Vasa previa is more common in assisted conceptions. If a low-lying placenta is observed during the routine anomaly ultrasound, a transvaginal ultrasound using color Doppler should be undertaken to look for vasa previa.[12]

TIMING AND MODE OF DELIVERY

There is a higher risk of preterm delivery in ART pregnancies because of intrinsic characteristics in a patient undergoing ART rather than the pregnancy. There are no specific recommendations for the prevention of preterm delivery in ART pregnancies.

Routine induction at term can be considered as there is a perceived risk of stillbirths in ART conceptions. If the patient desires, optimum maternal and fetal surveillance can be done and induction can be considered at 41 weeks. There is no evidence that elective induction of labor is needed at term in all ART conceptions.[3]

CONCLUSION

Antenatal care for ART pregnancies should be provided by a specialist with knowledge of obstetrics. High-order multiple pregnancies are the greatest risk of ART and selective reduction options should be discussed. There is some evidence of increased risk of congenital abnormalities and antenatal genetic and anatomic screening is recommended. Maternal surveillance for preeclampsia and preterm labor is needed in ART conceptions. An increased level of distress is a recognized feature in these pregnancies. Psychosocial care and counseling should be considered.[12]

REFERENCES

1. Nygren KG, Sullivan E, Zegers-Hochschild F, Mansour R, Ishihara O, Adamson GD, et al. International Committee for Monitoring Assisted Reproductive Technology (ICMART) World Report: Assisted Reproductive Technology 2003. Fertil Steril. 2011;95(7):2209-22, 2222.e1-17.
2. Chambers GM, Dyer S, Zegers-Hochschild F, de Mouzon J, Ishihara O, Banker M, et al. International Committee for Monitoring Assisted Reproductive Technologies World Report: Assisted Reproductive Technology, 2014. Hum Reprod. 2021;36(11):2921-34.
3. Richardson A, Taylor M, Teoh JP, Karasu T. Antenatal management of singleton pregnancies conceived using assisted reproductive technology. Obstet Gynecol. 2020;22(1):34-44.
4. Hansen M, Kurinczuk JJ, de Klerk N, Burton P, Bower C. Assisted reproductive technology and major birth defects in Western Australia. Obstet Gynecol. 2012;120(4):852-63.
5. Almasi-Hashiani A, Omani-Samani R, Mohammadi M, Amini P, Navid B, Alizadeh A, et al. Assisted reproductive technology and the risk of preeclampsia: an updated systematic review and meta-analysis. BMC Pregnancy Childbirth. 2019;19(1):149.
6. FOGSI-GESTOSIS-ICOG. Hypertensive Disorders in Pregnancy (HDP) Good Clinical Practice Recommendations 2019. [Online] Available from http://icogonline.org/images/stories/hdp_fogsi_gestosis_icog_gcpr_2019.pdf [Last accessed August, 2024].
7. Levron Y, Dviri M, Segol I, Yerushalmi GM, Hourvitz A, Orvieto R, et al. The 'immunologic theory' of preeclampsia revisited: a lesson from donor oocyte gestations. Am J Obstet Gynecol. 2014;211(4):383.e1-5.
8. Severino AI, Póvoa AM. Frozen embryo transfer and preeclampsia risk. J Gynecol Obstet Hum Reprod. 2021;50(9):102167.
9. Tandberg A, Klungsøyr K, Romundstad L, Skjaerven R. Pre-eclampsia and assisted reproductive technologies: consequences of advanced maternal age, interbirth intervals, new partner and smoking habits. BJOG. 2015;122(7):915-22.
10. Benlioglu C, Kalafat E, Sukur YE, Ozmen B, Sonmezer M, Atabekoglu CS. The association of adenomyosis with uteroplacental insufficiency and preeclampsia in women undergoing ICSI cycle. Fertil Steril. 2020;114(3):e211.
11. Cai S, Natarajan P, Chan JKY, Wong PC, Tan KH, Godfrey KM, et al. Maternal hyperglycemia in singleton pregnancies conceived by IVF may be modified by first-trimester BMI. Hum Reprod. 2017;32(9):1941-7.
12. Velez MP, Hamel C, Hutton B, Gaudet L, Walker M, Thuku M, et al. Care plans for women pregnant using assisted reproductive technologies: a systematic review. Reprod Health. 2019;16:9.

13. American College of Obstetricians and Gynecologists ACOG Committee opinion no. 553: multifetal pregnancy reduction. Obstet Gynecol. 2013;121(2 Pt 1): 405-10.
14. Chitayat D, Langlois S, Douglas Wilson R; SOGC Genetics Committee; CCMG Prenatal Diagnosis Committee. SOGC Genetics committee. Prenatal screening for fetal aneuploidy in singleton pregnancies. J Obstet Gynaecol Can. 2011;33(7):736-50.
15. Gameiro S, Boivin J, Dancet E, de Klerk C, Emery M, Lewis-Jones C, et al. ESHRE guideline: routine psychosocial care in infertility and medically assisted reproduction—a guide for fertility staff. Hum Reprod. 2015;30(11):2476-85.
16. Reefhuis J, Honein MA, Schieve LA, Correa A, Hobbs CA, Rasmussen SA. Assisted reproductive technology and major structural birth defects in the United States. Hum Reprod. 2009;24(2):360-6.
17. American College of Obstetricians and Gynecologists' Committee on Obstetric Practice. Committee opinion no 671: perinatal risks associated with assisted reproductive technology. Obstet Gynecol. 2016;128(3):e61-8.

CHAPTER 4

HELLP Syndrome

Girija Wagh

INTRODUCTION

HELLP syndrome, an intricate medical condition, emerges during pregnancy and the postpartum period. This acronym stands for hemolysis (H), elevated liver enzymes (EL), and low platelet count (LP).[1] The hallmark features of HELLP syndrome pose diagnostic challenges due to their potential overlap with preeclampsia.[2] While some evidence suggests that HELLP may represent an extreme manifestation of preeclampsia, the distinct nature of these conditions remains a subject of debate.[3] Notably, up to 20% of HELLP cases occur without antecedent hypertension or proteinuria.[4] The resolution of HELLP symptoms typically coincides with childbirth, yet maternal risks predominantly involve bleeding complications, including hepatic hemorrhage. Neonatal outcomes hinge on the gestational age at delivery, often occurring preterm, underscoring the urgency for timely intervention.

PREVALENCE

The prevalence of HELLP syndrome varies from 0.1% in pregnancies with normal blood pressure to 1% in pregnancies with preeclampsia without severe features.[4] The prevalence depends on the diagnostic criteria used.

RISK FACTORS

Previous history of HELLP syndrome is a significant risk factor for HELLP.[5] Certain genetic variants have been linked to an increased risk of HELLP syndrome in research studies. Unlike preeclampsia, being a primigravida is not a risk factor for HELLP syndrome. About >50% of patients affected are those who are multiparous.

PATHOGENESIS OF HELLP

The exact cause of HELLP syndrome is unclear. If it is a severe form of preeclampsia **(Table 1)**, it likely originates from the same source. If it is a separate condition, it may have a similar origin (like inadequate placentation), but for unknown reasons, it may follow a different pathway where liver inflammation and coagulation system activation exceed that in preeclampsia. Gestosis seems to be an appropriate term for HELLP taking this aspect into account.[6]

TABLE 1: PE diagnostic criteria and features of severe PE and superimposed PE.[7]

Blood pressure: SBP at ≥140 mm Hg and/or DBP ≥90 mm Hg on at least two occasions measured 4 hours apart in previously normotensive women and the new onset of one or more of the following:	
Proteinuria	>0.3 g in a 24-hour urine specimen Or Urine protein/creatinine ratio >0.3 (mg/mg) or 30 mg/mmol in a random urine sample Or Urine dipstick test ≥2+, if a quantitative measure is available
Platelets	<100,000/µL
Serum creatinine	>1.1 mg/dL (97.2 µmol/L) Or Doubling of the creatinine concentration in the absence of other renal disease
Liver transaminases	At least twice the upper limit of the normal concentrations of the local laboratory
Pulmonary edema	Clinical or radiological evidence
Cerebral or visual symptoms	New onset and persistent headaches not accounted for by alternate diagnoses and not responding to usual doses of analgesics, blurred vision, flashing lights or sparks, and scotomata
Superimposed preeclampsia	In women with chronic/preexisting hypertension: (1) New onset proteinuria; and/or (2) Significant end-organ dysfunction at 20+ weeks gestation
	In women with chronic/preexisting hypertension with proteinuria: (1) Worsening or resistant hypertension (especially acutely) in the last half of pregnancy or development of signs and symptoms of severe end of the disease

Note: If systolic BP is >160 mm Hg or diastolic BP is >110 mm Hg confirmation within minutes is sufficient and response to analgesia does not exclude the possibility of preeclampsia.
(BP: blood pressure; DBP: diastolic blood pressure; PE: preeclampsia; SBP: systolic blood pressure)

A subset of HELLP syndrome may be related to thrombotic microangiopathy caused by complement dysregulation (complement-mediated thrombotic microangiopathy). This may be treatable without immediate delivery of the baby. In one case report, a patient with severe early HELLP syndrome showed significant clinical improvement and complete normalization of laboratory parameters for 16 days after treatment with eculizumab, a targeted inhibitor of complement protein C5;[8] however, HELLP syndrome recurred after this period. This treatment was chosen based on the hypothesis that preeclampsia with severe features/HELLP syndrome is a systemic inflammatory disorder mediated by the complement cascade.[9] Pregnant individuals with pathogenic variants in complement regulatory proteins appear to be at increased risk for developing preeclampsia with severe features. Further research is needed to assess the potential benefits and risks before this clinical approach can be considered.

In fewer than 2% of patients with HELLP syndrome, the root cause seems to be linked to a deficiency in the fetal enzyme known as long-chain 3-hydroxyacyl CoA dehydrogenase (LCHAD). According to one case series, all six pregnancies involving fetuses with LCHAD deficiency resulted in severe maternal liver disease, manifesting as either HELLP syndrome or acute fatty liver of pregnancy (AFLP).[10] These complications are unlikely to be due to mere coincidence or solely due to maternal heterozygosity for LCHAD deficiency, as evidenced by three other pregnancies among these mothers with unaffected fetuses that proceeded without complications. In another case series, 79% (or 15 out of 19) of mothers carrying fetuses with LCHAD deficiency developed either AFLP or HELLP syndrome during their pregnancies.[11] While these findings contribute to our understanding of the pathogenesis of HELLP syndrome, it is important to note that screening for genetic variants associated with LCHAD deficiency does not play a role in the clinical management of patients with HELLP syndrome.

HELLP PATHOPHYSIOLOGY

Microangiopathy and activation of intravascular coagulation can explain all of the laboratory findings in HELLP syndrome.[12] Liver histology may show microvascular fibrin deposition, neutrophilic infiltrate, fatty infiltration, lobular necrosis, and periportal hemorrhage.[13] Even though kidney dysfunction is not a required condition for diagnosis, the kidney may experience microvascular dysfunction. This makes it more prone to ischemic damage from insufficient blood supply.[14]

CLINICAL PRESENTATION OF HELLP SYNDROME

HELLP syndrome, a severe form of preeclampsia, presents variably, with symptoms typically worsening over a short period.

Common Symptoms

The primary symptom is usually pain in the upper abdomen **(Fig. 1)**. This discomfort can be quite intense and constant, but it may also vary and exhibit a cramping nature. The pain can be pinpointed to the midepigastric region, the right upper quadrant, or beneath the sternum. Upon physical examination, these areas may also show signs of tenderness.

Many patients also experience nausea, vomiting, and generalized malaise, which can be mistaken for a nonspecific viral illness or viral hepatitis, especially if the serum aspartate aminotransferase (AST) and lactate dehydrogenase (LDH) levels are markedly elevated **(Fig. 1)**. In a substantial

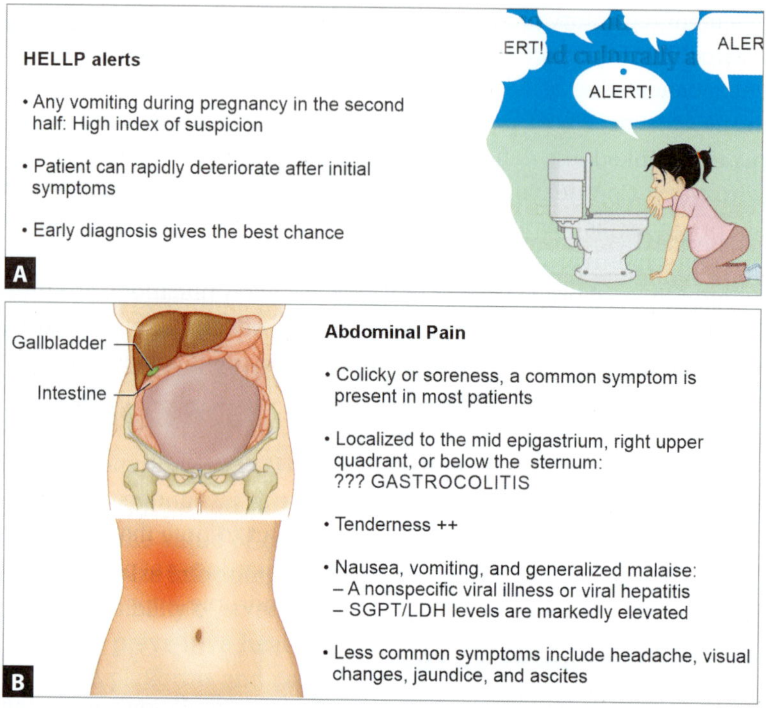

Fig. 1: Clinical presentation of HELLP. (A) HELLP alerts and (B) Abdominal pain. (HELLP: hemolysis, elevated liver enzymes, and low platelets; LDH: lactic dehydrogenase; SGPT: serum glutamic pyruvic transaminase)

series, the median level of AST was found to be 249 units/L, with a range spanning from 70 to 6,200 units/L. Similarly, the median level of LDH was 853 units/L, with the range extending from 560 to over 23,000 units/L **(Fig. 1)**.[15]

Physical Examination

Hypertension (blood pressure ≥140/90 mm Hg) and proteinuria are present in approximately 85% of cases. However, either or both may be absent in patients with HELLP. Thrombocytopenia-related bleeding (mucosal, hematuria, petechial hemorrhages, and ecchymosis) is an unusual presentation. The median platelet count was 57,000 cells/μL (range 7,000–99,000) in one large series.[15]

Severe Manifestations

Serious maternal morbidity may be present at initial presentation or develop shortly thereafter. Substantial hepatic bleeding (subcapsular or intraparenchymal liver hematoma) and rupture may lead to very severe pain, hypotension, and tachycardia; shoulder, chest, back, or neck pain; dyspnea or pain on inspiration; nausea/vomiting; and/or abdominal distention beyond that expected for the pregnant state. Some HELLP cases are complicated by eclampsia.

Other severe manifestations include placental abruption, acute kidney injury, pulmonary edema, and retinal detachment. Disseminated intravascular coagulation (DIC), if present, is usually associated with abruption, severe peripartum bleeding, or fulminant liver failure.

Gestational Age at Onset

Symptoms typically develop between 28 and 37 weeks of gestation, but onset in the late second trimester or at term/postpartum is also common. In a series including over 440 pregnancies complicated by HELLP, 70% of cases occurred before birth, approximately 80% of these occurred before <37 weeks, approximately 20% occurred before 28 weeks, and <3% occurred at 17–20 weeks.[15] In the 30% of cases that occurred postpartum, most were diagnosed within 48 hours after birth, but occasionally as long as 7 days; 80% had evidence of preeclampsia before birth. Why some cases of HELLP and preeclampsia develop postpartum is unknown and confusing since expulsion of the placenta initiates the resolution of the disease in most patients.

EVALUATION AND DIAGNOSIS OF HELLP SYNDROME

Diagnostic evaluation: In pregnant individuals with characteristic symptoms of HELLP (e.g., right upper quadrant/midepigastric pain, nausea, vomiting, and malaise) and/or new-onset hypertension in the second half of pregnancy or first postpartum week, laboratory tests are ordered to establish/exclude the diagnosis of HELLP. In rare cases of preeclampsia, severe persistent upper abdominal pain may precede laboratory abnormalities by several hours, so repeating the laboratory tests in 4–6 hours may be helpful unless another cause for the pain has been determined.

The laboratory work-up includes:

- Complete blood count
- Peripheral smear
- AST, alanine aminotransferase (ALT), and bilirubin
- Creatinine

An LDH level (as a marker for hemolysis) is needed to make a diagnosis of HELLP in some diagnostic protocols. For patients who exhibit increased levels of aminotransferases, haptoglobin, and LDH, coagulation studies that include tests for fibrinogen, prothrombin time, and activated partial thromboplastin time are prudent. The coagulation studies help to rule out AFLP in the absence of abruption and severe thrombocytopenia.

Diagnosis

The diagnosis of HELLP is based upon the presence of all of the laboratory abnormalities comprising its name [hemolysis with a microangiopathic blood smear (fragmented red blood cells, i.e., schistocytes and burr cells), elevated liver enzymes, and low platelet count] in a pregnant/postpartum patient. Pregnant/postpartum patients who have some of the typical laboratory abnormalities but do not have all of the laboratory criteria described below are considered to have partial HELLP (e.g., cases without hemolysis have been termed ELLP).

Laboratory Criteria for Diagnosis

Specifically, the laboratory parameters for the diagnosis of HELLP include hemolysis, which is the breakdown of red blood cells, elevated liver enzymes, indicating potential liver damage, and a low platelet count, suggesting a risk of excessive bleeding. These parameters not only aid in the diagnosis of HELLP syndrome but also help in determining the severity of the condition, thereby guiding the treatment decisions and providing an indication of maternal and fetal outcomes **(Table 2)**.

TABLE 2: Diagnosis criteria and classification of HELLP syndrome.

Tennessee classification	***The ACOG criteria***	***Mississippi classification***
Hemolysis, confirmed by at least two of the following: • Schistocytes and burr cells were observed in a peripheral smear • Serum bilirubin levels equal to or exceeding 1.2 mg/dL (20.52 μmol/L) • Serum haptoglobin levels ≤25 mg/dL or LDH levels at least twice the upper limit of normal (based on laboratory-specific reference ranges) • Severe anemia that is not related to blood loss • *Liver enzymes are elevated:* The levels of AST or ALT are at least double the maximum normal limit, as determined by specific laboratory reference ranges • *Platelet count is below the standard:* The count is <100,000 cells/μL	• LDH levels equal to or exceeding 600 IU/L • AST and ALT levels are more than twice the upper limit of normal • Platelet count <100,000 cells/μL	• *Class 1:* Platelet count ≤50,000 cells/μL, LDH levels >600 IU/L, and AST or ALT levels equal to or exceeding 70 IU/L • *Class 2:* Platelet count >50,000 but ≤100,000 cells/μL, LDH levels >600 IU/L, and AST or ALT levels equal to or exceeding 70 IU/L • *Class 3:* Platelet count >100,000 but ≤150,000 cells/μL, LDH levels >600 IU/L, and AST or ALT levels equal to or exceeding 40 IU/L
Necessitates the presence of all the following criteria	Mandates all the listed conditions be fulfilled	Severity of thrombocytopenia

(ACOG: American College of Obstetricians and Gynecologists; ALT: alanine aminotransferase; AST: aspartate aminotransferase; LDH: lactate dehydrogenase)

The Tennessee classification is what we use without the serum haptoglobin and LDH of more than 600 IU/L is used to categorize a severity. Low platelets as in the Mississippi classification are triggers to perform coagulation profile and choose anesthesia such as regional or general for birthing.

Case study 1: Gravida 2 Mrs ABC, abortion 1 with twin gestation with gestational hypertension (GHT) was referred to our institution for feeling uneasy and shortness of breath (SOB). She had a previous 9 weeks spontaneous miscarriage and had conceived with ovulation induction for perceived polycystic ovary syndrome (PCOS). She developed GHT at 35 weeks and was started on labetalol 100 mg twice daily. Her blood pressure records showed ranges from 140/100 to 130/90 mm Hg and she confirmed irregular intake of medications. She was referred to us at 38 weeks with SOB and was hospitalized and blood tests were sent. Her laboratory tests were done before admission representing HELLP but the action was not taken despite preeclampsia being diagnosed before referral to us. Significant deterioration of parameters is seen over 4 days when admitted to our center **(Table 3)**, such as a drop in platelets and a rise in LDH.

The woman was stabilized, massive transfusion protocol was initiated given microangiopathic hemolytic anemia, coagulopathy, and cardiac evaluation done. Electrolyte imbalance was corrected and a cesarean section was done after the correction of hyperkalemia **(Fig. 2)**.

- *Fragmented RBCs seen:* 8 PCVs + 6 FFPs + 4 RDP
- *Coagulation profile:* Deranged
- *Serum electrolytes:* Serum potassium: 6.1 mEq/L: Correction done (GI drip)
- *ECG:* Normal
- Cesarean section deferred till correction of hyperkalemia
- Cesarean done under GA after electrolyte imbalance was corrected
- No PPH
- *Intubated for:* 24 hours
- $MgSO_4$ continued for 24 hours

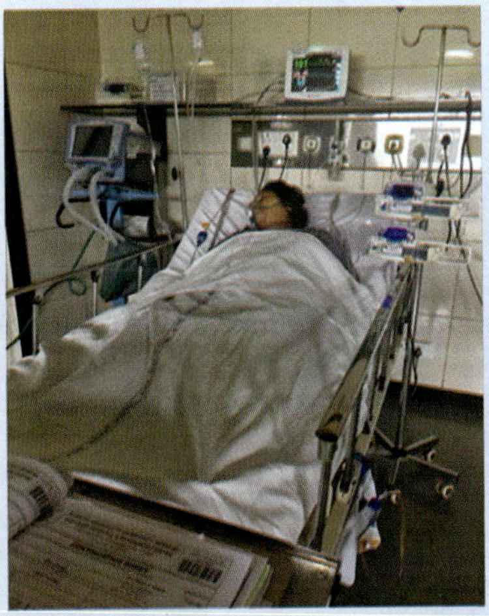

Fig. 2: HELLP: Cesarean section after stabilization. (ECG: electrocardiogram; FFP: fresh frozen plasma; HELLP: hemolysis, elevated liver enzyme levels, and low platelet levels; PCVs: packed cell volumes; RBCs: red blood cells; PPH: postpartum hemorrhage; RDP: random donor platelet)

TABLE 3: Case study of Mrs ABC: GHT evolving into PE/HELLP and critical hemolysis.

Date	*Hb (g/dL)*	*TLC*	*PLT*	*Urine*	*SAP*	*SGOT (IU/L)*	*SGPT*	*Bilirubin*	*BUN*	*Creatinine*	*LDH*
16/08	11.8	10,950	1.79	3+	418	42	42	0.67	44	Na	890
20/08	5.4	10,900	80,000	3+	420	195	155	0.6	43	0.89	1,990

Fragmented RBCs

Fragmented RBCs

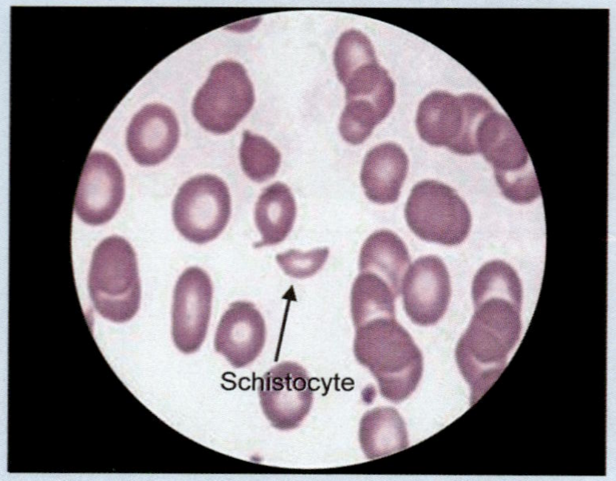

G2 A1 with twin gestation with GHT

Coagulogram	Before CS	After CS
PT seconds	9.0	12.2
PT control	10.6	
Laboratory range	9.6–13.4	
Mean N PT	11.6	
INR	0.78	1.05
Plasma fibrinogen	652	353
aPTT	26.5	27.9
Control	27.5	
aPTT range	26.6–35.5	

(BUN: blood urea nitrogen; aPTT: activated partial thromboplastin time; CS: cesarean section; GHT: gestational hypertension; Hb: hemoglobin; HELLP: hemolysis, elevated liver enzyme levels, and low platelet levels; INR: international normalized ratio; LDH: lactate dehydrogenase; PE: preeclampsia; PLT: platelet; PT: prothrombin time; RBCs: red blood cells; SGOT: serum glutamic-oxaloacetic transaminase; SGPT: serum glutamic pyruvic transaminase; TLC: total leukocyte count)

DIFFERENTIAL DIAGNOSIS OF HELLP SYNDROME

The differential diagnosis of HELLP syndrome involves several other disorders, and it is important to distinguish between them **(Fig. 3)**. The three major disorders: AFLP, thrombotic thrombocytopenic purpura (TTP), and pregnancy-related hemolytic uremic syndrome (HUS) usually pose a clinical dilemma **(Table 3)**. Other conditions such as gastroenteritis, hepatitis, appendicitis, gallbladder disease, lupus flare, antiphospholipid antibodies (APLA), pancreatitis, and nonalcoholic fatty liver disease can also contribute to confusion.

The distinguishing features of HELLP, TTP, HUS, and AFLP are shown in **Table 4**. There is also an overlap with preeclampsia with severe features **(Table 1)**, which may not be a separate disease.

In HELLP, angiopathy (including thrombotic microangiopathy and microangiopathic hemolytic anemia) and liver dysfunction are marked, and the magnitude of hypertension is not highly correlated with the level of angiopathy and liver dysfunction. By contrast, most cases of severe preeclampsia have severe hypertension; thrombocytopenia and liver dysfunction, although present, are not as markedly abnormal as in HELLP.

Given the striking similarity in clinical and histologic features, it may not be feasible to establish an accurate diagnosis. Moreover, it is important to note that HELLP syndrome can manifest simultaneously with these conditions. Additionally, severe acute respiratory syndrome coronavirus 2 (SARS-CoV-2) infection during pregnancy has been associated with a significant increase in the odds of preeclampsia with severe features, eclampsia, and HELLP.

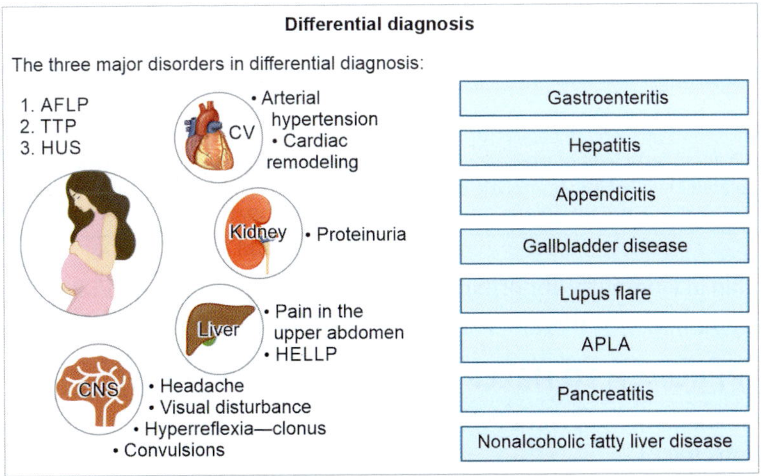

Fig. 3: Differential diagnosis of HELLP. (AFLP: acute fatty liver of pregnancy; APLA: antiphospholipid antibodies; CNS: central nervous system; CV: cardiovascular; HELLP: hemolysis, elevated liver enzyme levels, and low platelet levels; HUS: hemolytic uremic syndrome; TTP: thrombotic thrombocytopenic purpura)

TABLE 4: The distinguishing features of HELLP, TTP, HUS, and AFLP.

Condition	*Thrombotic thrombocytopenic purpura*	*Hemolytic uremic syndrome*	*Hemolysis, elevated LFT tests, and low PLT*	*Acute fatty liver of pregnancy*
Abdominal pain	++	++	++	++
Low ADAMST13 activity	+/++	–	±	?
Anemia	++	++	+	+
Elevated lactic dehydrogenase	++ very high values	++ very high values	++	+/++
Elevated transaminases	±	±	++	++
Fever	+	–	–	+
Headache or visual disturbances	++	–	++	±
Hypertension	+/++	++	++	–
Jaundice	–	–	+	+
Nausea and vomiting	++	++	++	++
Proteinuria	+ and hematuria	++	++	–
Thrombocytopenia	++	++	++	+
von Willebrand factor	++	++	–	??
Hypoglycemia	++	++	++	++
+Prevalence of findings in affected patients				

(AFLP: acute fatty liver of pregnancy; HELLP: hemolysis, elevated liver enzyme levels, and low platelet levels; HUS: hemolytic uremic syndrome; LFT: liver function test; PLT: platelets; TTP: thrombotic thrombocytopenic purpura)

Overlap in laboratory abnormalities between COVID-19 and HELLP syndrome can complicate the diagnosis of HELLP in patients infected with the virus.

APPROACH TO HELLP SYNDROME MANAGEMENT

The management of HELLP syndrome is a multifaceted process, as depicted in **Flowchart 1**.

- *Optimal care setting:* For patients diagnosed with HELLP syndrome, it is imperative to provide care in a tertiary medical facility equipped with advanced maternal and neonatal intensive care units (ICUs) necessary to handle serious complications such as liver rupture, acute kidney injury, and DIC.

Flowchart 1: Management of women with HELLP.

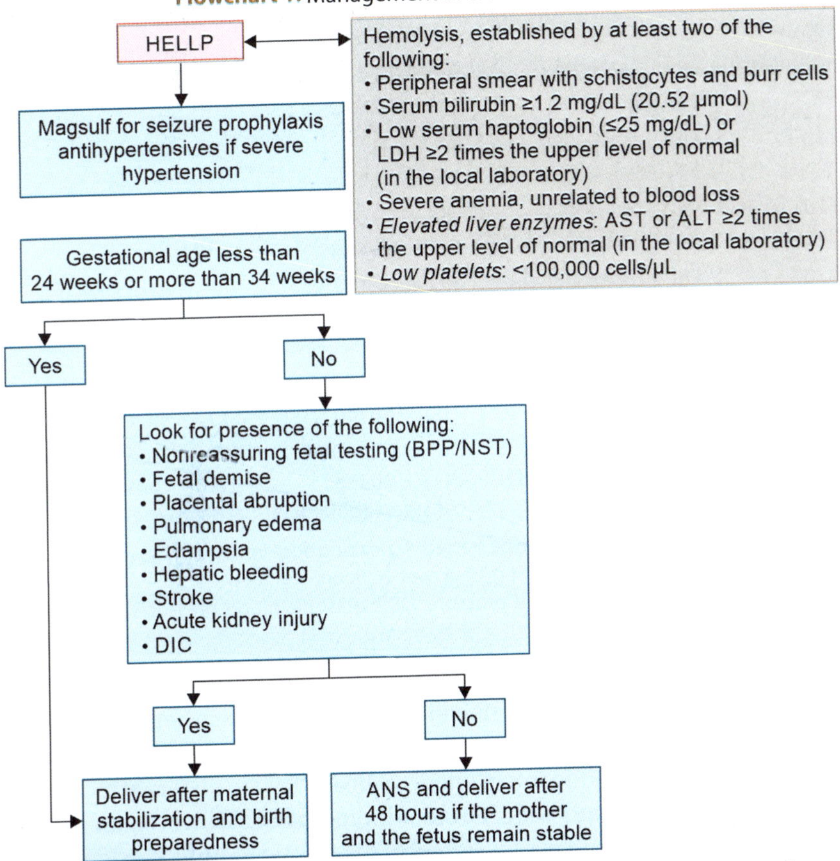

(ALT: alanine aminotransferase; ANS: antenatal steroids; AST: aspartate aminotransferase; BPP: biophysical profile; DIC: disseminated intravascular coagulopathy; LDH: lactose dehydrogenase; NST: nonstress test)

- *Managing severe hypertension:* In cases of severe hypertension, it is essential to administer antihypertensive medications[16] immediately to mitigate the risk of cerebrovascular accidents. The protocol for managing hypertension in HELLP syndrome aligns with that established for preeclampsia **(Table 5)**.

Dexamethasone in HELLP Syndrome

The role of dexamethasone in managing HELLP syndrome has been explored in various studies, yielding different results. Some early research suggested that dexamethasone could expedite the improvement of maternal laboratory and clinical parameters. However, more robust randomized, double-blind, placebo-controlled trials did not confirm these benefits. A meta-analysis that

TABLE 5: Management of severe hypertension (Ready Reckoner).

Time (minutes)	*Labetalol oral*	*Nifedipine*	*Labetalol IV*
0	200 mg	10 mg	20 mg
10	SBP ≥160 or DBP ≥110 wait	BP check	SBP ≥160 or DBP ≥110—40 mg
20	SBP ≥160 or DBP ≥110 wait	SBP ≥160 or DBP ≥110—20 mg	SBP ≥160 or DBP ≥110—80 mg
30	SBP ≥160 or DBP ≥110 labetalol IV/ nifedipine 20 mg	BP check	SBP ≥160 or DBP ≥110—80 mg
40	BP check	SBP ≥160 or DBP ≥110—20 mg	SBP ≥160 or DBP ≥110—80 mg
50	SBP ≥160 or DBP ≥110 additional AHT	SBP ≥160 or DBP ≥110—20 mg/ consider labetalol IV	SBP ≥160 or DBP ≥110—consider other antihypertensive

Note: Magnesium sulfate infusion to be started: 4 g loading dose in 100 mL NS over 10 minutes or in the infusion pump at a rate of 1 g/hour over 24 hours.

(AHT: antihypertensive; BP: blood pressure; DBP: diastolic blood pressure; SBP: systolic blood pressure; IV: intravenous)

included 11 trials with 550 participants compared corticosteroid treatment to placebo or no treatment in HELLP Syndrome cases.[17] The findings did not convincingly show a reduction in maternal death, severe maternal morbidity, or perinatal/infant death with steroid administration. However, an average increase in platelet count was observed in the steroid group.

An additional randomized trial involving 132 patients compared dexamethasone to placebo.[18] The study found no significant differences in the recovery time for platelet counts and AST levels, or in the incidence of complications. As a result, the effectiveness of dexamethasone in treating HELLP Syndrome remains unclear. It is crucial for healthcare professionals to consider the most recent and comprehensive research when making treatment decisions for conditions, such as HELLP syndrome.

Magnesium Sulfate in the Management of HELLP Syndrome

Research has established a correlation between hemolysis and magnesium deficiency, with significant decreases in serum magnesium levels observed in those with hemolytic anemia. This deficiency is also seen in liver diseases, influencing body magnesium content and increasing liver enzymes. A link has been found between thrombocytes and magnesium levels, suggesting serum magnesium is involved in the function of platelets.[19]

Once a diagnosis of HELLP is made, expectant management is recommended by 34 weeks gestation, with regular comprehensive metabolic panels, complete blood count, urinalysis, and coagulation profiles. Magnesium sulfate therapy and hypertensive management are highly recommended if the diagnosis is made within the time frame of 24–34 weeks. Magnesium sulfate is the first treatment given to treat HELLP syndrome, causing cerebral vasodilation to reduce ischemia in blood vessels, therefore reducing hypertension.

HELLP syndrome is associated with endothelial injury, deposition of fibrin in the lumen of blood vessels, and increased platelet activation with platelet consumption. In pregnancies affected by preeclampsia, concentrations of magnesium were decreased and those of platelet-activating factor (PAF) were increased. Increased magnesium intake has increased the synthesis of prostacyclin, suggesting that exogenous magnesium should be one of the first courses of action to treat preeclampsia. Hypertensive conditions are a common complication seen in pregnancies, affecting both maternal and fetal health. When unchecked, they can progress to chronic hypertension, preeclampsia, and HELLP syndrome. A decreased concentration of magnesium has many detrimental effects on the body such as hypertension and vasoconstriction. Experimental studies have shown that supplementation of magnesium in hypertensive pregnancies resulted in decreased blood pressure. The etiology linking the role of PAF is not fully understood and further investigation is warranted. Given the current understanding of intravenous magnesium utilization in clinical practice, it would be beneficial for research to explore the introduction of dietary magnesium in mothers at various gestational ages to determine the point in the timeline that introduction is most crucial.

ADDITIONAL HELLP SYNDROME COMPLICATIONS, IMAGING, AND INTERVENTIONS

Patients may also develop other complications associated with HELLP syndrome, such as DIC, pulmonary edema, or acute kidney injury. These conditions require management with standard medical treatments.

Liver Imaging in HELLP

For patients presenting with intense symptoms indicative of hepatic complications, timely imaging is crucial, regardless of the extent of elevation in liver enzyme levels. Initial evaluations can be conducted using bedside ultrasound [focused assessment with sonography in trauma (FAST)], followed by a thorough ultrasound assessment. If necessary, computed tomography (CT) or magnetic resonance imaging (MRI) scans can be used for more informed clinical decision-making.

Hepatic Hemorrhage

In the event of hepatic bleeding, which may be self-contained or lead to liver rupture and subsequent intraperitoneal hemorrhage, immediate medical intervention is critical. This is particularly vital to prevent life-threatening outcomes for both the mother and the fetus. Treatment involves volume resuscitation and blood transfusions. Once the patient's condition is stable, and any severe anemia or coagulopathy has been treated, urgent cesarean delivery may be warranted.

Disseminated Intravascular Coagulation

This complication necessitates clinical diagnosis and prompt management.

Pulmonary Edema

Pulmonary edema is a possible complication during pregnancy and the peripartum period and warrants appropriate fluid and transfusion protocols and monitoring and astute evaluation.

Acute Kidney Injury

This condition may arise during pregnancy. Magnesium sulfate is administered upon admission to the labor and delivery unit and continued for 24 hours postpartum to prevent maternal seizures and provide fetal/neonatal neuroprotection for pregnancies under 32 weeks of gestation.

THERAPEUTIC PLASMA EXCHANGE

While not beneficial for HELLP patients, it is the primary treatment for TTP. Distinguishing between HELLP and TTP is challenging due to similar presentations of microangiopathic hemolysis and thrombocytopenia.

BIRTHING PROTOCOLS FOR HELLP SYNDROME

Optimal Timing for Delivery

The definitive treatment for HELLP syndrome is delivery. Once the mother's condition is stable, delivery is advised for pregnancies at 34 weeks or later, or earlier if there are significant complications. In pregnancies under 34 weeks without critical issues, delivery may be postponed for a maximum of 48 hours to allow for the administration of antenatal corticosteroids, enhancing neonatal outcomes. If the fetus has not yet reached a viable stage poststeroid treatment, immediate delivery becomes necessary.

Management Expectations

Expectant management is generally discouraged for HELLP syndrome at any stage of pregnancy. Although some cases have shown laboratory improvements with this approach, there is no substantial proof that it betters perinatal outcomes when compared to prompt delivery following antenatal corticosteroids.

Use of Antenatal Corticosteroids

Administering antenatal corticosteroids and delaying delivery for up to 48 hours can be beneficial for neonates in pregnancies under 34 weeks. This advantage, however, must be carefully balanced with the potential maternal risks associated with prolonging the pregnancy. Betamethasone for fetal lung development is not recommended for pregnancies at or beyond 34 weeks.

Preferred Birthing Method

The default preference is for vaginal delivery unless there are clear reasons for a cesarean, such as standard obstetric indications or hepatic bleeding. In cases of HELLP syndrome with hepatic bleeding, a cesarean route of birth is the recommended course of action.

Pain Management and Anesthesia

Due to the risk of thrombocytopenia and coagulation issues, neuraxial anesthesia may not be viable for labor and delivery. Intravenous opioids or inhalation analgesics can offer pain relief without increasing the risk of bleeding. The use of local anesthesia for episiotomy or perineal repair does not have any contraindications.

Cesarean Birth and Surgical Assessment

Thrombocytopenia management during birth aligns with the protocols for preeclampsia with severe features. A cesarean birth facilitates direct assessment of bleeding sources and volumes. Caution has to be adopted at the time of any surgical intervention such as cesarean birth or episiotomy and if a peritoneal tear or cervical tear occurs through rule out for hematoma is essential. Cesarean section should be done swiftly, maintaining the placental perfusion, minimal tissue handling, and ensuring that the blood vessels and sinusoids below the rectus muscle are not blindly teased. This can cause retromuscular hematoma and a lot of clinical heartaches later for the patient and the doctors.

Immediate Postdelivery Care

Postpartum patients experiencing hepatic bleeding warrant the same level of care. Surgical procedures are necessary for those with unstable hemodynamics or ongoing bleeding. This also applies to cases where there is an increase in pain or the hematoma size is growing, as observed in serial ultrasounds. In hemodynamically stable patients, hepatic artery embolization can be considered as an initial treatment option.

POSTPARTUM MANAGEMENT OF HELLP SYNDROME

Postpartum Presentation

Symptoms and signs of HELLP syndrome, such as subcapsular hematoma and liver rupture, may manifest for the first time after childbirth. The management protocol aligns with that for HELLP-diagnosed predelivery, minus the need to consider fetal well-being.

Maternal Care Considerations

Patients in critical condition or those at high risk of serious complications should be considered for transfer to an ICU rather than a standard postpartum ward. Conditions warranting intensive care include potential or actual liver rupture, severe liver failure, DIC, acute renal failure, extensive transfusion requirements, transfusion-related lung injury, and cardiac issues such as ischemia or cardiomyopathy. Placental abruptions and intrauterine devices (IUDs) are usually taken for granted and are an endpoint of a serious disease pathogenesis that should be remembered. This is so because placental separation causes the thromboplastin to enter the maternal circulation initiating the DIC cascade and IUD implies >70% placental separation.[20]

Supportive Measures

Supportive Care Encompasses (Fig. 4)

- Oxygen support and ventilation assistance (e.g., supplemental oxygen or mechanical breathing support)
- Sedation and pain management
- Hemodynamic stabilization using agents, such as vasopressors
- Rigorous monitoring
- Fluid balance via IV fluids or diuretics
- Nutritional support
- Prevention of stress ulcers
- Prophylaxis against venous thromboembolism

Laboratory Monitoring

Postdelivery, lab results may initially deteriorate, with platelet counts typically dropping by 40% daily, hematocrit levels decreasing, and liver enzyme levels rising.[21] It is advisable to conduct lab tests every 12 hours during the initial postpartum days.[22] Testing can cease once laboratory values show clear signs of stabilization, barring complications from HELLP or hemorrhage.

Recovery Indicators

By Day 4 postpartum, barring complications, a rising platelet count, and falling LDH levels are expected. Recovery is indicated by a platelet count

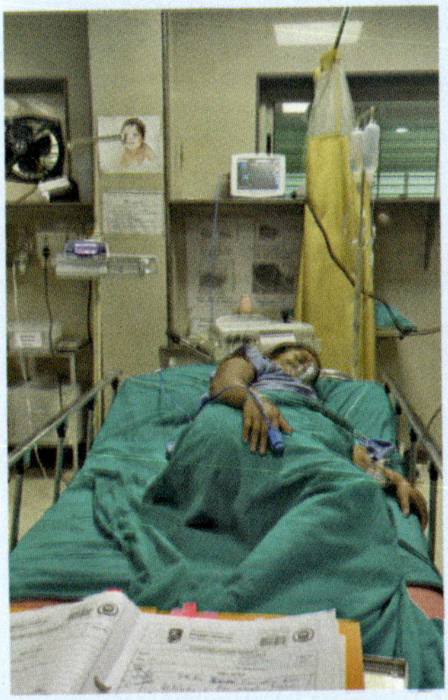

$MgSO_4$: IV regimen: 4–6 g/l00 mL
NS: 15–20 minutes
2 g/hour: Intrapartum and 12–24 hours postpartum
40 g/1 L RL@50 mL/hour. Infusion pump

Fluids: Foley/fluids l00 mL/hour: *Pulmonary edema:* Frusemide 40 mg IV: XRC/maternal ECHO

Monitor vitals: SpO_2/RR/PR/BP/reflexes
Crossmatch: PCV asks for MTP: Inform blood bank
Platelets <40,000/μL: 6–10 U: before delivery/CS

Continuous fetal monitoring

Oxytocin induction if ripe cervix or GA 30 weeks or > CS: <30 weeks/unripe cervix/OBS indication

Anesthesia: Epidural preferred: platelets less or reducing trend; general anesthesia
Minimize the risk of hematoma at the bladder flap/muscle layer. Consider subfascial drain.

Fig. 4: Management of HELLP an overview. (BP: blood pressure; CS: cesarean section; GA: gestational age; HELLP: hemolysis, elevated liver enzyme levels, and low platelet levels; IV: intravenous; MTP: massive transfusion protocol; NS: normal saline; PR: pulse rate; RL: Ringer's lactate; RR: respiratory rate; XRC: X-ray chest)
Note: Ideal nursing position is slightly propped up with lateral recumbent and respectful maternal care it is warm cover despite gadgets attached.

exceeding 100,000 cells/μL by Day 6 postpartum or within 72 hours from the lowest platelet count recorded. Occasionally, platelet counts can rebound to levels between 413,000 and 871,000 cells/μL.[23]

Further Considerations

Should platelet counts continue to decline and LDH levels rise beyond Day 4 postpartum, alternative diagnoses to HELLP syndrome should be explored. In cases of severe HELLP, such as those involving DIC, platelet counts below 20,000 cells/μL, renal impairment, and ascites, recovery may be protracted.[24] These patients are at heightened risk for pulmonary edema and acute renal failure.

PERINATAL AND LONG-TERM OUTCOMES IN HELLP SYNDROME

Maternal Prognosis

While the prognosis for patients with HELLP syndrome is generally favorable, there is a potential for severe complications. These may include:

- Hemorrhagic events
- DIC

- Placental abruption
- Acute renal injury
- Pulmonary edema
- Subcapsular liver hematoma
- Retinal detachment
- Intracerebral hemorrhage
- In extreme cases, mortality

Such complications are notably more prevalent in early-onset forms of HELLP syndrome. Nonetheless, the long-term renal function remains unaffected by HELLP syndrome, and no chronic liver issues persist postrecovery from hepatic complications.

Fetal and Neonatal Outcomes

The neonatal and long-term health of the newborn is closely linked to the gestational age at delivery and the infant's birth weight. Premature births are frequent, with associated risks such as fetal growth restriction and placental abruption being primary factors in perinatal mortality. Early-onset HELLP syndrome carries a significantly adverse prognosis.

Recurrence in Future Pregnancies

The recurrence rate of HELLP syndrome stands at approximately 4% among individuals who were normotensive before its onset.[25] Nonetheless, these individuals face a heightened risk for other placenta-related obstetric issues. In subsequent pregnancies, a considerable number of patients may develop hypertensive conditions, including HELLP syndrome, preeclampsia, GHT, or eclampsia.

Preventive Measures and Contraceptive Choices

Currently, no therapeutic interventions have been proven to prevent the recurrence of HELLP syndrome. However, prophylactic administration of low-dose aspirin during the second and third trimesters is commonly recommended to mitigate the risk of preeclampsia. Consultation with a healthcare provider, especially considering the increased thrombotic risk associated with hormonal methods in women with a history of HELLP syndrome. Nonhormonal options such as barrier methods, IUDs, or sterilization may be more appropriate. It is essential to discuss and determine the most suitable contraceptive method based on individual circumstances.

CONCLUSION

- *HELLP syndrome:* It is a severe pregnancy-related disorder marked by hemolysis (H), elevated liver enzymes (EL), and low platelet count (LP). It poses diagnostic challenges due to potential overlap with preeclampsia.

- *Prevalence and risk factors:* The prevalence varies from 0.1% in pregnancies with normal blood pressure to 1% in pregnancies with preeclampsia. Risk factors include a previous history of HELLP syndrome and certain genetic variants.
- *Pathogenesis and pathophysiology:* The exact cause of HELLP syndrome is unclear. It may be related to thrombotic microangiopathy caused by complement dysregulation or a deficiency in the fetal enzyme known as LCHAD.
- *Clinical presentation:* Symptoms typically develop between 28 and 37 weeks of gestation but can also occur at term/postpartum. Common symptoms include upper abdominal pain, nausea, vomiting, and generalized malaise.
- *Evaluation and diagnosis:* The diagnosis is based on the presence of all laboratory abnormalities comprising its name in a pregnant/postpartum patient. Different classification systems exist, including the Tennessee classification, the American College of Obstetricians and Gynecologists (ACOG) criteria, and the Mississippi classification.
- *Differential diagnosis:* It is important to distinguish HELLP syndrome from other disorders such as AFLP, TTP, pregnancy-related complement-mediated thrombotic microangiopathy (CM-TMA), and systemic lupus erythematosus.
- *Management:* Management involves several steps, including treatment of severe hypertension, hepatic imaging, management of hepatic bleeding, and addressing other complications. Delivery is the primary treatment for HELLP syndrome.
- *Postpartum management:* All symptoms and signs of HELLP syndrome can first appear in the postpartum period. The management approach is similar to that of HELLP diagnosed before birth.
- *Perinatal and long-term aspects:* The neonatal and long-term prognoses are most strongly associated with gestational age at birth and birth weight. The risk of recurrent HELLP syndrome is about 4% for patients who were normotensive before the onset of the syndrome.
- *Prevention and contraception:* There is no evidence that any therapy prevents recurrent HELLP syndrome. However, low-dose aspirin is often prescribed during the second and third trimesters in future pregnancies to reduce the risk of preeclampsia. Hormonal methods may not be recommended for women with a history of HELLP syndrome due to the increased risk of blood clots. Barrier methods, IUDs, or sterilization may be suitable options.

REFERENCES

1. Weinstein L. Syndrome of hemolysis, elevated liver enzymes, and low platelet count: a severe consequence of hypertension in pregnancy. Am J Obstet Gynecol. 1982;142(2):159-67.

2. Yeasmin S, Nazneen R, Akhter S, Jahan N. HELLP syndrome: a diagnostic dilemma. North Int Med Coll J. 2015;7(1):87.
3. Gupte S, Wagh G. Preeclampsia-eclampsia. J Obstet Gynaecol India. 2014;64(1):4-13.
4. Sibai BM, Taslimi MM, El-Nazer A, Amon E, Mabie BC, Ryan GM. Maternal-perinatal outcome associated with the syndrome of hemolysis, elevated liver enzymes, and low platelets in severe preeclampsia-eclampsia. Am J Obstet Gynecol. 1986;155(3):501-7.
5. van Oostwaard MF, Langenveld J, Schuit E, Papatsonis DN, Brown MA, Byaruhanga RN, et al. Recurrence of hypertensive disorders of pregnancy: an individual patient data meta-analysis. Am J Obstet Gynecol. 2015;212(5):624.e1-17.
6. Wagh G, Wagh R. Hypertensive disorders: delivery management. In: Sharma A (Ed). Labour Room Emergencies. Singapore: Springer Verlag; 2020. pp. 63-76.
7. American College of Obstetricians and Gynecologists, Task Force on Hypertension in Pregnancy. Hypertension in pregnancy. Report of the American College of Obstetricians and Gynecologists' Task Force on Hypertension in Pregnancy. Obstet Gynecol. 2013;122 (5):1122-31.
8. Burwick RM, Feinberg BB. Eculizumab for the treatment of preeclampsia/HELLP syndrome. Placenta. 2013;34(2):201-3.
9. Burwick RM, Feinberg BB. Complement activation and regulation in preeclampsia and hemolysis, elevated liver enzymes, and low platelet count syndrome. Am J Obstet Gynecol. 2022;226(2S):S1059-70.
10. Treem WR, Rinaldo P, Hale DE, Stanley CA, Millington DS, Hyams JS, et al. Acute fatty liver of pregnancy and long-chain 3-hydroxyacyl-coenzyme A dehydrogenase deficiency. Hepatology. 1994;19(2):339-45.
11. Ibdah JA, Bennett MJ, Rinaldo P, Zhao Y, Gibson B, Sims HF, et al. A fetal fatty-acid oxidation disorder as a cause of liver disease in pregnant women. N Engl J Med. 1999;340(22):1723-31.
12. Perez Botero J, Reese JA, George JN, McIntosh JJ. Severe thrombocytopenia and microangiopathic hemolytic anemia in pregnancy: a guide for the consulting hematologist. Am J Hematol. 2021;96(12):1655-65.
13. Barton JR, Riely CA, Adamec TA, Shanklin DR, Khoury AD, Sibai BM. Hepatic histopathologic condition does not correlate with laboratory abnormalities in HELLP syndrome (hemolysis, elevated liver enzymes, and low platelet count). Am J Obstet Gynecol. 1992;167(6):1538-43.
14. Ye W, Shu H, Yu Y, Li H, Chen L, Liu J, et al. Acute kidney injury in patients with HELLP syndrome. Int Urol Nephrol. 2019;51(7):1199-206.
15. Sibai BM, Ramadan MK, Usta I, Salama M, Mercer BM, Friedman SA. Maternal morbidity and mortality in 442 pregnancies with hemolysis, elevated liver enzymes, and low platelets (HELLP syndrome). Am J Obstet Gynecol. 1993;169(4):1000-6.
16. Chapter 21 Hypertensive Disorders in Pregnancy: Clinical Approach. In: Wagh GNK (Ed). Manual for Obstetrics & Gynecology Practitioners. New Delhi: Jaypee Brothers Medical Publishers; 2015. pp. 179-90.
17. Woudstra DM, Chandra S, Hofmeyr GJ, Dowswell T. Corticosteroids for HELLP (hemolysis, elevated liver enzymes, low platelets) syndrome in pregnancy. Cochrane Database Syst Rev. 2010;9:CD008148.

18. Fonseca JE, Méndez F, Cataño C, Arias F. Dexamethasone treatment does not improve the outcome of women with HELLP syndrome: a double-blind, placebo-controlled, randomized clinical trial. Am J Obstet Gynecol. 2005;193(5):1591-8.
19. Chawla N, Shah H, Huynh K, Braun A, Wollocko H, Shah NC. The role of platelet-activating factor and magnesium in obstetrics and gynecology: is there crosstalk between pre-eclampsia, clinical hypertension, and HELLP syndrome? Biomedicines. 2023;11(5):1343.
20. Wagh G. Antepartum haemorrhage: Practical Approach towards Evaluation and Management. In: Studd J, Lin tan S, Chervenak FA (Eds). Current Progress in Obstetrics and Gynaecology. New Delhi: Tree Life Media; 2022. pp. 95-119.
21. Martin JN Jr, Blake PG, Perry KG Jr, McCaul JF, Hess LW, Martin RW. The natural history of HELLP syndrome: patterns of disease progression and regression. Am J Obstet Gynecol. 1991;164(6 pt 1):1500-9; discussion 1509-13.
22. Gestational Hypertension and Preeclampsia: ACOG Practice Bulletin, Number 222. Obstet Gynecol. 2020;135(6):e237-60.
23. Neiger R, Contag SA, Coustan DR. The resolution of preeclampsia-related thrombocytopenia. Obstet Gynecol. 1991;77(5):692-5.
24. Martin JN Jr, Blake PG, Lowry SL, Perry KG Jr, Files JC, Morrison JC. Pregnancy complicated by preeclampsia-eclampsia with the syndrome of hemolysis, elevated liver enzymes, and low platelet count: how rapid is postpartum recovery? Obstet Gynecol. 1990;76(5 Pt 1):737-41.
25. Malmström O, Håberg SE, Morken NH. Probability and outcomes of second pregnancy after HELLP syndrome in the first: a population-based registry study. Acta Obstet Gynecol Scand. 2020;99(9):1206-13.

CHAPTER 5

Etiopathogenesis of HDP

Gorakh G Mandrupkar, Swati Bhargava

INTRODUCTION

Hypertensive disorders of pregnancy (HDP) constitute a spectrum of conditions that can have significant implications for maternal and fetal health and pose risks to the mother and the fetus. It encompasses a range of conditions such as gestational hypertension, preeclampsia, eclampsia, and chronic hypertension with superimposed preeclampsia. Understanding the etiopathogenesis of these disorders is crucial for effective management and prevention. This chapter covers the multifactorial origins, pathophysiological mechanisms, and risk factors associated with hypertensive disorders during pregnancy.

DEFINITIONS AND CLASSIFICATION

Hypertensive disorders of pregnancy are classified into several categories, each with distinct characteristics:

- *Gestational hypertension:* Elevated blood pressure (≥140/90 mm Hg) after 20 weeks of gestation without the presence of proteinuria or other systemic features.
- *Preeclampsia:* Characterized by hypertension and proteinuria after 20 weeks of gestation, it may also present with systemic features such as renal insufficiency, liver dysfunction, neurological complications, and fetal growth restriction.
- *Eclampsia:* The occurrence of seizures in a woman with preeclampsia, which can lead to significant morbidity and mortality.
- *Chronic hypertension:* Present before pregnancy or diagnosed before 20 weeks of gestation, which may also be complicated by superimposed preeclampsia.

Understanding these classifications is essential for diagnosing and managing hypertensive disorders effectively **(Flowchart 1)**.

EPIDEMIOLOGY

Hypertension is the most common medical disorder occurring during pregnancy, complicating 5–10% of all pregnancies globally.[1] Prevalence rates can vary significantly by region and are influenced by maternal age, race, and socioeconomic factors. The rising prevalence of obesity and chronic diseases contributes to the increasing incidence of HDP in many populations.

Flowchart 1: Etiopathogenesis of hypertensive disorders of pregnancy.

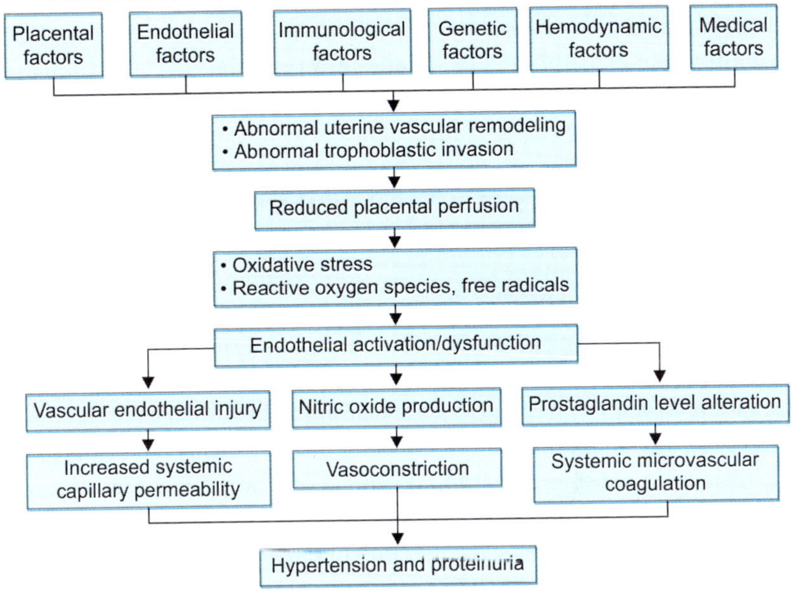

RISK FACTORS

Several risk factors predispose individuals to HDP:

- *Demographic factors:* Advanced maternal age, particularly women over 35 years old, are at higher risk.
- *Obesity:* Body mass index (BMI) over 30 kg/m^2 significantly increases the likelihood of developing HDP.
- *Chronic conditions:* Preexisting hypertension, diabetes, and renal disease are notable contributors.
- Increased risk of metabolic syndrome and hyperhomocysteinemia.
- *Past obstetric history:* Previous abruption, previous preeclampsia, and prior stillbirth.
- *Multiple gestations:* The presence of twins or higher-order multiples elevates the risk of hypertensive disorders.
- *Family history:* A familial history of preeclampsia or hypertension increases susceptibility.
- Women conceived with assisted reproductive techniques.
- Pregnancies with male fetuses are at slightly higher risk.[2]
- *Ethnicity:* Certain ethnic groups, including African American and Hispanic populations, exhibit higher incidences of hypertensive disorders.

PATHOPHYSIOLOGY

The etiopathogenesis of HDP is complex and involves a combination of genetic, environmental, and immunological factors.

Placental Factors

In normal placentation, spiral arterioles undergo changes in decidua basalis and endovascular trophoblasts invade and remodel the endothelial and muscular lining of the arterioles to enlarge the diameter of the vessels.

The placenta plays a central role in the development of hypertensive disorders. Abnormal placentation is a hallmark of preeclampsia, characterized by inadequate remodeling of maternal spiral arteries, leading to reduced blood flow to the placenta.

Impaired Trophoblastic Invasion

Proper trophoblastic invasion of maternal spiral arteries is crucial for normal placentation. In HDP, this invasion is often inadequate, leading to insufficient remodeling of maternal blood vessels leading to lesser external diameter of the vessels, less than 50% than the normal placenta. This results in narrow, high-resistance arteries and impaired placental perfusion.[3] This impaired remodeling leads to placental ischemia and subsequent release of factors that contribute to endothelial dysfunction and hypertension.

Placental Ischemia and Hypoxia

The impaired remodeling leads to placental ischemia, triggering a cascade of pathological events.

Ischemic placentas produce several bioactive factors, including soluble fms-like tyrosine kinase 1 (sFlt-1) and antiangiogenic factors. sFlt-1 acts as a decoy receptor for vascular endothelial growth factor (VEGF), leading to decreased angiogenesis and exacerbation of hypertension.[4]

Endothelial Dysfunction

Endothelial dysfunction is a critical event in the pathogenesis of HDP. It is characterized by a reduced ability of blood vessels to dilate and an increased tendency for thrombosis.

Altered Nitric Oxide Production

In a normal pregnancy, endothelial nitric oxide synthase (eNOS) activity increases to promote vasodilation. In preeclampsia, eNOS expression and activity are often reduced, leading to diminished nitric oxide availability, increased vascular resistance, and elevated blood pressure.[5]

Increased Levels of Endothelin-1

Endothelin-1, a potent vasoconstrictor, is often elevated in women with HDP. This increase contributes to heightened vascular tone and further promotes endothelial dysfunction and thus exacerbates hypertension.[6]

Immune System Dysregulation

The maternal immune response is pivotal in the development of hypertensive disorders. In normal pregnancies, there is an adaptive immune response promoting tolerance to the fetus, while in HDP, this balance is disrupted.

Increased Inflammatory Cytokines

Women with preeclampsia often exhibit elevated levels of proinflammatory cytokines such as tumor necrosis factor-alpha (TNF-α), interleukin-6 (IL-6), and IL-1β. These cytokines contribute to systemic inflammation, endothelial dysfunction, and vascular damage leading to increased vascular permeability.[7]

Immune Cell Activation

Abnormal activation of immune cells, particularly monocytes and macrophages, plays a significant role in the pathogenesis of HDP. These cells release inflammatory mediators that perpetuate vascular dysfunction and hypertension.[8]

Genetic Factors

Genetics significantly influence susceptibility to hypertensive disorders. Various candidate genes involved in angiogenesis, endothelial function, and immune responses have been implicated.

Genetic Polymorphisms

Several gene polymorphisms (single nucleotide polymorphisms SNPs) have been associated with an increased risk of developing HDP, including those involved in the renin-angiotensin system and endothelial function, such as the angiotensinogen gene, (*eNOS* gene) and various cytokines.[9]

Epigenetic Modifications

Epigenetic modifications, including deoxyribonucleic acid (DNA) methylation and histone modification, can influence gene expression and have been implicated in the pathogenesis of HDP, highlighting the complex interactions between genetics and environmental factors.[10]

Maternal Factors

Several maternal characteristics and preexisting conditions can contribute to the development of hypertensive disorders during pregnancy.

Obesity and Metabolic Syndrome

Obesity is associated with chronic low-grade inflammation, insulin resistance, and altered vascular function, all of which can predispose women to HDP. Elevated adipokine levels in obese individuals can further disrupt endothelial function and increase vascular resistance.[11]

Chronic Stress and Psychosocial Factors

Psychosocial stressors and chronic mental health conditions can also influence pregnancy outcomes. Increased stress levels can activate the sympathetic nervous system, endothelial dysfunction and alter blood pressure regulation.[12]

Hemodynamic Changes

Pregnancy induces significant hemodynamic changes that can predispose women to hypertension. The increased plasma volume and cardiac output are usually compensated by a decrease in systemic vascular resistance.

Altered Vascular Reactivity

During normal pregnancy, there is a decrease in systemic vascular resistance. In women with hypertensive disorders, there is an impaired ability to adapt to the hemodynamic changes of pregnancy, leading to increased vascular resistance and elevated blood pressure.[13]

Neurohormonal Activation

Increased activity of the renin-angiotensin-aldosterone system (RAAS) has been observed in women with HDP, contributing to sodium retention, increased blood volume, and elevated blood pressure. This activation contributes to sodium retention, increased blood volume, and elevated blood pressure.[14]

CONCLUSION

The etiopathogenesis of HDP is multifactorial, involving a complex interplay between genetic, environmental, and physiological factors. A thorough understanding of these mechanisms is essential for the effective management and prevention of these disorders. Ongoing research is vital to uncover further insights into the pathophysiology of HDP, which may ultimately lead to improved screening, prevention, and therapeutic strategies for affected women. By addressing these challenges, healthcare providers can help reduce the burden of hypertensive disorders during pregnancy and promote healthier outcomes for mothers and their infants.

REFERENCES

1. Hutcheon JA, Lisonkova S, Joseph KS. Epidemiology of pre-eclampsia and the other hypertensive disorders of pregnancy. Best Pract Res Clin Obstet Gynaecol. 2011;25(4):391-403.

2. Jaskolka D, Retnakaran R, Zinman B, et al. Fetal sex and maternal risk of preeclamsia/eclampsia: a systematic review and meta-analysis. BJOG. 2017;124(4):553-60.
3. Zhang J, Wei J, Xu Y, Wang Y. Abnormal trophoblastic invasion in preeclampsia. Journal of Clinical Investigation, 2021;131(3):e135926.
4. Roberts JM, Gammill HS, von Dadelszen, P. Endothelial dysfunction in preeclampsia. Circulation. 2018;138(12):1247-60.
5. Lisonkova S, Joseph KS. Incidence of preeclampsia: risk factors and outcomes. Obstetrics & Gynecology. 2013;122(5):1148-55.
6. Meyer MR, Kaciroti N, Herington JL, Banz J, Jones JH, Black JE. Endothelin-1 and its role in pregnancy. Trends in Cardiovascular Medicine. 2020;30(7):348-57.
7. Gonzalez JS, Langer JC, Sacks GP, McLaughlin MC. Cytokine patterns in preeclampsia. American Journal of Reproductive Immunology. 2017;77(2):e12600.
8. Nicolas D, Hertig A, Tchernitchin N, Kacem S, Boudjema A. Role of macrophages in the pathogenesis of preeclampsia. Frontiers in Immunology. 2019;10:308.
9. Bergström S, Järvefelt H, Lehtinen M, Niskanen E. Genetic risk factors for preeclampsia. International Journal of Molecular Sciences. 2018;19(3):646.
10. Harris LK, Yung HW, Burton GJ. Epigenetics in preeclampsia: impact on placentation and pregnancy outcome. Clinical Epigenetics. 2017;9:116.
11. Davis BA, Qiu C, Williams MA. Obesity and pregnancy: a review of the pathophysiology and implications for management. American Journal of Obstetrics and Gynecology. 2019;220(1):21-31.
12. Hobel CJ, Goldstein A, Barrett-Connor E. Psychosocial stress and pregnancy outcome. Clinical Obstetrics and Gynecology. 2008;51(2): 333-48.
13. Petersen JK, Klemm H, Schmitz R. Hemodynamic changes in normal and hypertensive pregnancies. Journal of Clinical Hypertension. 2019;21(3): 384-91.
14. Smith SK, Williams SM, Leung TM. The role of the renin-angiotensin system in preeclampsia. Frontiers in Pharmacology. 2020;11:346.

CHAPTER 6 Overview of ART Law

Geetendra Sharma, Riddhi Desai

INTRODUCTION

The Assisted Reproductive Technology (Regulation) Act was passed on December 20, 2021, by an Act of Parliament.[1] It is a major milestone Act that provides a framework to regulate the practice of assisted reproductive technology (ART) in India. The Act addresses ethical, legal, and social issues associated with ART and aims to protect the rights of infertile couples and surrogate mothers while also providing guidelines for accreditation and monitoring of ART clinics.

This overview will help infertility specialists navigate the key provisions of the Act and include them in their clinical practice.

Global Perspective of ART Regulation

The regulatory landscape for ART has evolved significantly since the birth of the world's first in vitro fertilization (IVF) baby in 1978.[2] UK's Human Fertilization and Embryology Act of 1990 marked the first regulatory attempt, which was later updated in 2009.[3] The US has the American Society for Reproductive Medicine (ASRM) guidelines in place.[4] Many European countries have banned gamete donation and surrogacy.

PRESSING NEED FOR REGULATORY ACT IN INDIA

In India, although the Indian Council of Medical Research (ICMR) has issued guidelines, there remains a significant gap in regulation, leading to concerns about potential unethical practices.[5] With the mushrooming of private ART clinics and banks, there is a pressing need for comprehensive guidelines to prevent commercialization and ensure ethical standards. Before the Assisted Reproductive Technology (Regulation) Act, the responsibility of enforcing ICMR guidelines fell to state accreditation authorities. The new Act aims to safeguard the rights of infertile couples and surrogate mothers, providing financial security to oocyte donors with insurance coverage for 12 months. Surrogacy, though banned in several European countries, is permitted in India, attracting international couples seeking these services.

MERITS AND SHORTCOMINGS OF THIS ACT

The six chapters of the Act cover various aspects of ART, including technical terms and processes involved in ART and how to regulate ART clinics and banks. It also covers research in assisted reproduction and establishes national and state ART and surrogacy boards to implement and oversee compliance. A national ART registry will facilitate data collection, research, and policy development. The Act includes provisions for preimplantation genetic diagnosis and ethical embryo sex selection. It mandates the collection of personal information from gamete donors and surrogate mothers to ensure transparency and targeted delivery of benefits.

The Act guarantees that children born through ART are legally recognized as the biological children of the couple and details penalties for noncompliance. It also protects doctors and authorities acting in good faith and provides flexibility for future amendments based on technological and social changes.

Despite its merits, the Act has notable shortcomings. It lacks detailed guidelines on the qualifications and experience required for ART clinic staff, such as gynecologists and embryologists. The regulation of adoption, often a subsequent step for couples failing ART, is not addressed, nor are the specifics of surrogacy contract disputes. These gaps are critical given the influx of international surrogacy seekers.

KEY PROVISIONS

Establishment of Regulatory Bodies

National Board

The Act establishes the National Assisted Reproductive Technology and Surrogacy Board. This body is responsible for formulating policies, guidelines, and codes of conduct for ART clinics and banks, ensuring uniformity and adherence to ethical practices.

State Boards

Each state is required to establish its own State Assisted Reproductive Technology and Surrogacy Board. These boards are responsible for the implementation and monitoring of the Act's provisions at the state level, ensuring compliance with the National Board's guidelines.

Registration of ART Clinics and Banks

All ART clinics and banks must be registered under the Act to provide ART services. Registration requires clinics and banks to meet specific criteria, including infrastructure, equipment, and staff qualifications, as outlined by the National Board.

National Registry

The Act mandates the creation of a National ART and Surrogacy Registry. This centralized database will maintain records of all registered ART clinics and banks, facilitating transparency and accountability in ART services.

Regulation of ART Services

Assisted reproductive technology services include a range of procedures such as IVF, intrauterine insemination (IUI), and other assisted reproductive technologies aimed at treating infertility.

The Act requires the establishment of standard protocols for ART procedures. These protocols ensure the safety, efficacy, and ethical conduct of ART treatments, reducing the risk of malpractice and ensuring high-quality care.

Prohibited Practices

This includes sex selection, cloning, and the use of ART for commercial surrogacy or other nonpermitted purposes.

Protection of Donor and Surrogate Rights

Donor Rights

The Act outlines the rights and duties of gamete donors (sperm and egg donors). It mandates informed and voluntary consent for donation and prohibits the sale or purchase of gametes. Donors are entitled to receive compensation for their expenses but not for the gametes themselves.

Surrogate Rights

The Act safeguards the interests of the surrogates, preventing exploitation and ensuring they receive proper medical care and compensation. Surrogates must provide informed consent and are entitled to health insurance coverage for a specified period.

Rights of Children Born Through ART

Children born through ART procedures are granted the same rights as those born through natural conception. This includes the right to information about their biological origins once they reach 18 years of age. ART clinics and banks are required to maintain the confidentiality of donor identities. However, this information must be accessible to the child upon reaching adulthood, ensuring transparency, and respecting the child's right to know their biological origins.

Ethical Considerations

The Act mandates the establishment of ethical committees in ART clinics that oversee the ethical aspects of ART services, ensuring compliance with the guidelines and addressing any ethical dilemmas that may arise. The Act strictly prohibits practices such as sex selection, cloning, and any form of commercial exploitation of ART services. Violating these provisions can result in severe penalties, including fines and imprisonment.

Grievance Redressal

Complaints Committees

The Act establishes mechanisms for the redressal of grievances related to ART services. Complaints committees at the national and state levels are responsible for addressing complaints and ensuring fair resolution.

Appeal Process

Individuals aggrieved by the decisions of the complaint's committees can appeal to higher authorities, ensuring a fair and transparent process for grievance redressal.

Penalties and Offences

The Act outlines specific penalties for various offenses, including operating an unregistered ART clinic, using ART services for nonpermitted purposes, and violating the rights of donors, surrogates, or children born through ART. Penalties range from fines to imprisonment, depending on the severity of the offense.

Sex-Selective Technology

Clinics, banks, or agents are prohibited from advertising or promoting sex-selective ART in any form, including online. Violators face imprisonment from 5 to 10 years, a fine between 10 and 25 lakh rupees, or both.

General Offences and Penalties

Prohibited actions:

- Abandon or exploit children born through ART
- Sell or trade human embryos or gametes
- Import human embryos or gametes
- Exploit commissioning couples, donors, or women
- Transfer human embryos to males or animals
- Sell embryos or gametes for research
- Use intermediaries to acquire gametes

Penalties: For the first offense, fines range from 5 to 10 lakh rupees. For repeated offenses, penalties include imprisonment from 3 to 8 years and fines from 10 to 20 lakh rupees.

Punishment for Unspecified Violations

Violations not explicitly covered by specific penalties in the Act will incur fines and imprisonment as per the provisions for general offenses.

Legal Procedures

Only complaints from the National or State Board, or authorized officers, can initiate legal action. Offenses are tried by courts no lower than a Metropolitan Magistrate or Judicial Magistrate of the First Class.

Cognizance of Offences

All offenses under the Act are cognizable and bailable, meaning that they can be arrested without a warrant and bail can be granted.

IMPLICATIONS AND SPECIAL CONSIDERATIONS FOR FERTILITY SPECIALISTS

Compliance with Regulations

Fertility specialists must ensure that their clinics are registered under the Act. This involves meeting the criteria set by the National and State Boards, including infrastructure, equipment, and staff qualifications. Compliance with the standard protocols established by the National Board is essential. This ensures the safety and efficacy of ART procedures, reducing the risk of malpractice and enhancing patient outcomes.

Patient Counseling

Providing thorough counseling and discussing the procedures, potential risks, success rates, and alternative options with patients helping them make informed decisions is essential. Infertility and ART treatments can be emotionally challenging for patients. Psychological support should be given and, when necessary, refer patients to counseling services to help them cope with the stress and emotional impact.

Ethical Practice and Addressing Ethical Dilemmas

Obtaining informed and voluntary consent from patients, donors, and surrogates is crucial. Gynecologists must discuss the procedures, potential risks, success rates, and legal and ethical aspects of ART services. They must protect the rights of donors, surrogates, and children born through ART. They must maintain confidentiality, provide proper medical care, and ensure fair compensation.

Gynecologists should establish ethical committees within their clinics to oversee the ethical aspects of ART services. These committees can guide us on complex ethical issues, ensuring compliance with the Act's provisions and addressing any ethical dilemmas that may arise. Regular ethical training for all staff involved in ART procedures is crucial. The team should be well-versed in the ethical guidelines and standards set by the Act, promoting a culture of ethical practice within the clinic.

Documentation and Reporting

Accurate documentation and reporting of ART procedures are essential. Maintaining detailed records of all procedures, including patient information, treatment protocols, and outcomes, ensuring transparency and accountability.

Collaboration with Regulatory Bodies

Gynecologists need to collaborate with regulatory bodies at the national and state levels. This includes staying updated with changes in policies, guidelines, and protocols, and ensuring compliance with the Act's provisions. Maintaining accurate records and documentation is essential. All required information should be properly documented and reported to the relevant authorities, facilitating transparency and accountability.

Ensuring Quality Care and Patient-centered Care

Providing high-quality care to patients undergoing ART procedures is paramount. Clinics should be equipped with the necessary infrastructure, equipment, and skilled staff to deliver safe and effective treatments. Gynecologists should engage in continuous professional development, staying updated with advancements in ART technologies and techniques. This ensures the provision of cutting-edge treatments and enhances patient outcomes. Treatment plans should be tailored for each patient considering their medical history, preferences, and individual needs. This approach enhances patient satisfaction and improves the likelihood of successful outcomes.

Screening and Selection of Donors

Gamete donors should undergo thorough medical and psychological screening. This includes assessing the donor's medical history, genetic background, and psychological well-being to minimize risks and ensure the safety of the recipient and the resulting child. Donors must provide informed and voluntary consent for the donation. The donation process, potential risks, and the donor's rights and responsibilities should be explained to ensure that donors make informed decisions.

Surrogacy Arrangements

When involving surrogates in ART procedures, gynecologists must ensure that surrogacy arrangements comply with the ethical guidelines set forth by the Act. This includes obtaining informed consent, ensuring fair compensation, and protecting the surrogate's health and well-being. Comprehensive medical care should be provided to surrogates including proper prenatal and postnatal care, with regular check-ups, monitoring, and support throughout the pregnancy and postpartum period.

CHALLENGES IN IMPLEMENTATION OF THE ACT

Implementing the Act presents considerable obstacles. The task of registering numerous ART clinics and banks, along with ensuring adherence to the Act's provisions, is complex and demanding. Each state is required to create tailored regulations. Legal disputes in surrogacy agreements, especially with international clients, may arise. Enforcing restrictions on the cross-border transfer of gametes and embryos is also challenging. Additionally, establishing and maintaining the national ART registry, and utilizing it effectively for policy development, will necessitate significant effort and cooperation among various stakeholders.

CONCLUSION

The Assisted Reproductive Technology (Regulation) Act, 2021, is a major step taking in the right direction aiming at regulating ART practices in India, offering essential protections for infertile couples and surrogate mothers. The Act introduces numerous benefits, such as improved regulation, ethical guidelines, and data collection mechanisms. However, its success will depend on addressing existing limitations and navigating implementation challenges effectively. Proper enforcement is vital to uphold ethical standards and safeguard the interests of all parties involved in assisted reproduction.

For fertility specialists, understanding and integrating the Act's key provisions into clinical practice is crucial for promoting ethical practices. This involves complying with registration requirements, following standardized protocols, securing informed consent, and ensuring the rights of donors, surrogates, and children are protected, all while delivering comprehensive, patient-centered care. Collaboration with regulatory bodies, meticulous documentation, and continuous professional development are essential for maintaining compliance with the Act and improving patient outcomes. By fostering ethical practices and high standards of care, gynecologists and infertility specialists can help ensure that ART services remain safe, effective, and accessible, ultimately enhancing patient well-being and advancing the field of reproductive medicine in India.

REFERENCES

1. Gazette of India. Ministry of Law and Justice (Legislative D). The Assisted Reproductive Technology (Regulation) Act, 2021 (No. 42 of 2021).
2. Kamel RM. Assisted reproductive technology after the birth of Louise Brown. J Reprod Infertil. 2013;14(3):96-109. PMID: 24163793; PMCID: PMC3799275.

3. Agrawal R, Burt E, Homburg R. Time-line in HFEA Developments and Regulatory Challenges: 20 years of Overseeing Fertility Practices and Research in the UK. J Obstet Gynaecol India. 2013;63(6):363-9. doi: 10.1007/s13224-013-0494-z. Epub 2013 Dec 11. PMID: 24431680; PMCID: PMC3889279.
4. Jamwal VDS, Yadav AK. The Assisted Reproductive Technology (Regulation) Act, 2021: A Step in the Right Direction. Indian J Community Med. 2023;48(1):4-6. doi: 10.4103/ijcm.ijcm_169_22. Epub 2022 Dec 8. PMID: 37082392; PMCID: PMC10112746.
5. National Guidelines for Accreditation, Supervision & Regulation of ART Clinics in India, ICMR. Available online on https://main.icmr.nic.in/.

CHAPTER 7

DNA Fragmentation Testing

N Sanjeeva Reddy, Radha Vembu

INTRODUCTION

The male factor influences the success of infertility treatment. Normally, it is assessed by semen analysis done in a standard laboratory. The semen tests are based on the World Health Organization (WHO) criteria which include analysis of semen volume, sperm concentration, total sperm count, motility, and morphology. However, the sensitivity of semen analysis for assessing the fertility potential is low; so, sperm evaluation based on conventional semen analysis may not predict the embryonic potential, pregnancy, and miscarriage rates. This has led to the emergence of sperm deoxyribonucleic acid (DNA) fragmentation (SDF).

There is an increase in the prevalence of infertility with 1 in 6 couples suffering from infertility. Among them, 50% is attributable to male factor.[1] In men with unexplained infertility, the pregnancy rate is very low even though semen analysis is normal. So alternate tests for sperm function were considered and among them, SDF and reactive oxygen species (ROS) are easily reproducible tests.

Normally, the sperm DNA undergoes a unique and highly specific process to ensure a compact and stable nuclear chromatin. The sperm nuclear matrix undergoes complete decondensation so that the entire genome is anchored to a single structure within the base of the tail is called the *nucleus annulus*. The degree of condensation of chromatin affects epididymal maturation, transfer of genetic information to the oocyte, and embryo development.

The decondensation of the sperm nucleus occurs in the oocyte and allows the formation of the male pronucleus. The sperm introduce the reproducing and microtubular organization elements of centrosome and sperm-specific phospholipase C zeta induces calcium oscillation which stimulates oocyte activation and early embryonic development.[2] SDF is hypothesized to contribute to the "late paternal effect" which affects embryo development after fertilization from day 2–5.

Sperm DNA damage can originate from the testes or during transit through the male reproductive system. The sperms acquire progressive motility and fertilizing capacity while passing through the epididymis where the epithelium promotes normal secretion and absorption function and hence an appropriate microenvironment for the maturation of sperms. However, during this transit, oxidative stress (OS) can affect the sperm chromatin. SDF is induced by defective maturation and abortive apoptosis in the testes or by OS throughout the male genital tract.

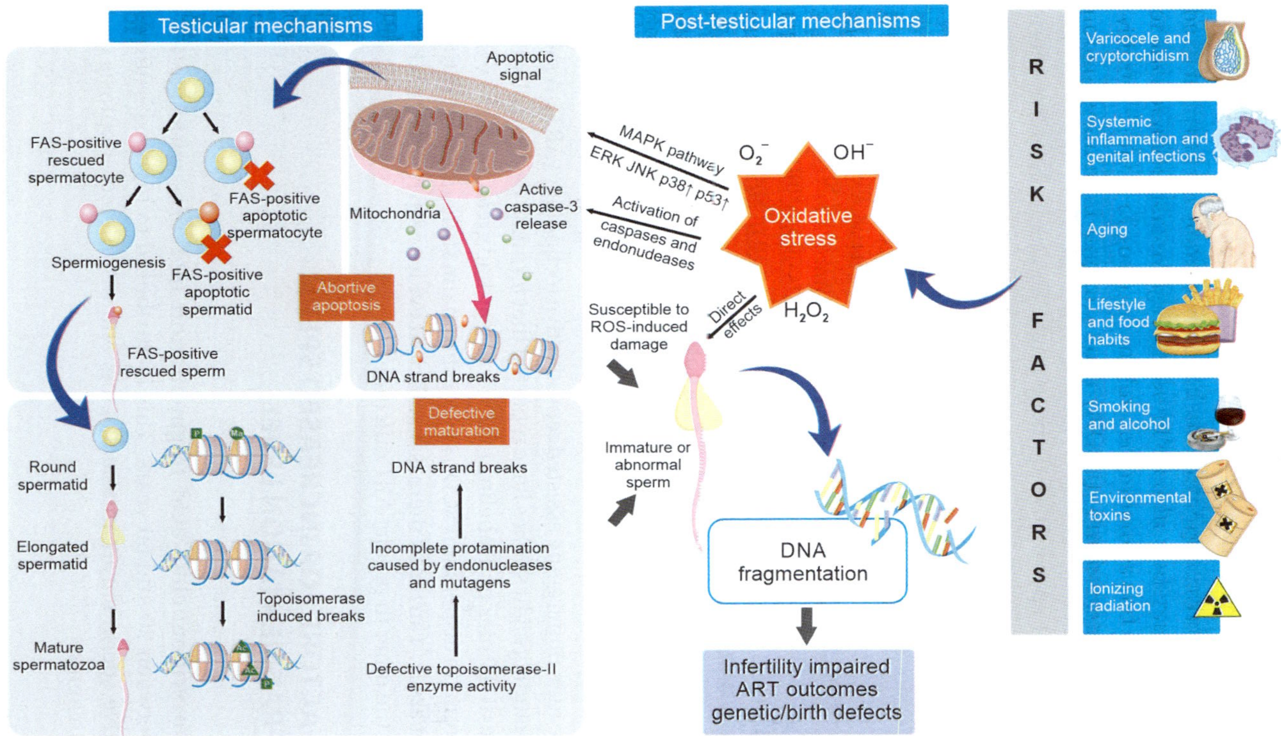

Fig. 1: Overview of the origins of SDF.[4] (ART: assisted reproductive technology; DNA: deoxyribonucleic acid; ERK: extracellular signal-regulated kinase; JNK: c-Jun N-terminal kinase; MAPK: mitogen-activated protein kinase; ROS: reactive oxygen species; SDF: sperm deoxyribonucleic acid fragmentation)

PREVALENCE OF SPERM DNA FRAGMENTATION

Among the general population, 1–4% of men have a DNA fragmentation index (DFI) >30%. With increase in SDF, 64% of men have decreased reproductive potential.

MECHANISM OF SPERM DNA DAMAGE (FIG. 1)

The mechanism for sperm DNA damage might be due to defective sperm chromatin packaging. During spermatogenesis, chromatin is compacted through histone exchange with transitional proteins and protamines which is facilitated by endogenous nuclease topoisomerase II, creating DNA breaks to reduce torsional stress for histone disassembly and chromatin packaging. If these breaks are not repaired, chromatin packaging may be impaired leading to defective maturation of sperms with increased SDF in ejaculate. Apoptosis ensures that no defective germ cells differentiate into spermatozoa, but the failure of this process leads to the accumulation of sperms expressing apoptotic markers in the ejaculated semen.

Excess of ROS can activate the apoptotic pathway and increase SDF. In addition, indirectly through by-products of lipid peroxidation such as malondialdehyde (MDA) and 4-hydroxynonenal (4HNE) result in SDF.

Sperm deoxyribonucleic acid fragmentation is emerging as a novel marker for infertile men undergoing assisted reproductive technology (ART). A meta-analysis including eight studies have reported that terminal deoxynucleotidyl transferase dUTP nick end labeling (TUNEL) assay had greater accuracy than sperm chromatin dispersion (SCD), sperm chromatin structure assay (SCSA), and Comet assay.[3] Currently there is insufficient evidence to recommend one assay over the other to predict ART outcome.

RISK FACTORS FOR INCREASED SPERM DNA FRAGMENTATION LEVEL

Aging

Sperm deoxyribonucleic acid fragmentation increases with age and doubles between 20 and 60 years. This is attributed to high exposure to OS, defective sperm chromatin packaging, and disordered apoptosis that occurs with aging.

Varicocele

It is seen in 35–40% of men presenting with infertility. Testicular hyperthermia and OS affect the membrane function and sperm damage due to an increase in ROS due to the retrograde flow of renal and adrenal metabolites. A meta-analysis involving 240 patients with 176 normal controls, showed significantly higher sperm DNA damage compared to normal control men, and varicocelectomy improved sperm DNA integrity.[5] SDF test is recommended before varicocele repair in patients with grade 2–3 varicocele who have normal semen parameters and in grade 1 varicocele with borderline or abnormal semen parameters.[6]

- Male genital tract infection—increases ROS production.
- Cigarette smoking—negatively impacts SDF due to tobacco metabolites, such as nicotine, cadmium, lead, and benzopyrene.
- Alcohol—can increase SDF and cause apoptosis.
- Diabetes mellitus—has high levels of SDF due to OS in addition to the generation of advanced glycation and products. There is associated dysfunction of the hypothalamopituitary gonadal axis along with disruption of sympathetic innervation and increased inflammatory response.
- Thyroid dysfunction can affect the testicular function and redox status.
- *Obesity:* Obese men have higher levels of OS and SDF. this might be due to increased scrotal temperature, endocrine imbalance, and chronic systemic inflammation.
- Ionizing radiation.
- Electromagnetic waves from cell phones increase mitochondrial ROS production and DNA adduct formation causing DNA damage.[7]
- Chemotherapy
- Malignancy—testicular cancer and other malignancies that might increase SDF secondary to the associated endocrine alterations of OS.
- Leukocytospermia
- *Endocrine disruptors:* Exposure to bisphenol A used in plastics and resins.
- Exposure to gonadotoxins, such as organophosphate, carbamate, and insecticides.
- Studies have shown SDF in ejaculated sperm is higher than in testicular sperms suggesting that SDF may originate from post-testicular environment. In a study, it was shown that SDF in testicular sperm was lower than in ejaculated sperm (8.3% vs. 40.7%), clinical pregnancy rate (CPR) (51.9% vs. 40.2%), and live birth rate (LBR) (46.9% vs. 26.4%) was better with testicular sperms with lower miscarriage rate, (10% vs. 34.3%) hence favoring testicular sperms over ejaculated sperms.[8]

NEED FOR TESTING SPERM DNA FRAGMENTATION

- Sperm DNA damage can lead to
- Impaired fertilization, slow early development of an embryo, reduced implantation, and increased miscarriage.
- Birth defects in offspring in animal studies.
- Childhood cancers—due to oxidative damage secondary to paternal smoking.

METHODS OF MEASURING SPERM DNA FRAGMENTATION (TABLE 1)

Sperm deoxyribonucleic acid fragmentation tests are generally classified into direct and indirect assays. In direct assays, the extent of SDF is measured by

TABLE 1: Comparison of various SDF assays.[4]

Assay	*Principle*	*Type of damage detected*	*Pros*	*Cons*
TUNEL	Labeling of free break ending 3-OH DNA	SSB/DSB	• High sensitivity and reliability • Minimal inter-observer variability • Evaluation by both fluorescent micros-copy and flow cytometry • Analysis of both fresh and frozen samples	• Protocols and thresholds are still not standardized • Expensive equip-ment and trained personnel are required
Comet	Single-cell electrophoretic separation	SSB and/or DSB	• High sensitivity • Correlation with semen parameters • Possibility to dis-criminate between SSB and DSB	• Poor repeatability. • High interob-server variability • Variable protocols and thresholds • Time-consuming • Evaluation of a low number of cells • Appropriate imaging software required
SCSA	Evaluation of DNA integrity by using the metachromatic acridine orange	SSB/DSB	• Simultaneous exam-ination of a large number of cells • Highly repeatability • Analysis of frozen or fresh samples	• Commercial kits are not available • Expensive equip-ment and trained personnel are required
SCD or Halo-sperm test	Evaluation of the dispersed chro-matin ("halo") after lysing treatment	SSB/DSB	• Commercial kits are available • Repeatable and consistent results in 45 minutes • No expensive equipment required • Easy to perform	Interobserver vari-ability

(DNA: deoxyribonucleic acid; DSB: double strand break; SCD: sperm chromatin dispersion; SCSA: sperm chromatin structure assay; SDF: sperm deoxyribonucleic acid fragmentation; SSB: single strand break; TUNEL: terminal deoxynucleotidyl transferase dUTP nick end labeling)

using probes and dyes directly as in Comet assay and TUNEL assay. In indirect assays, both the existing breaks and the susceptibility of DNA to denaturation which occurs more commonly in fragmented DNA are measured as in SCSA, and SCD tests.

Aniline blue staining, chromomycin A3 staining, and toluidine blue staining are the assays that measures the level of chromatin compaction. However, tests that measure DNA fragmentation are preferred, such as Comet assay, TUNEL assay, SCSA, and SCD assay. Several studies have attempted to identify the cutoff value of the SDF test to predict the outcome. Although there is no unanimous consensus, studies have taken a cutoff value of 20–30% depending on the assay method.

COMMON SPERM DNA FRAGMENTATION TESTS (FIGS. 2 AND 3)

Preparation of Semen Sample

- A neat semen sample should be used for SDF testing.
- A fixed ejaculatory abstinence before the collection of semen sample is required.
- In the majority of places, density gradient centrifugation was the common preparation technique for intracytoplasmic sperm injection (ICSI) before

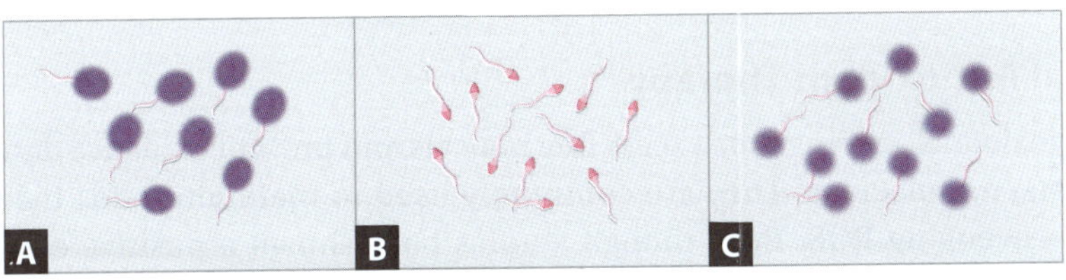

Figs. 2A to C: Sperm chromatin dispersion assay. (A) Intact sperm deoxyribonucleic acid (DNA); (B) Highest DNA fragmentation; (C) Moderate DNA fragmentation.

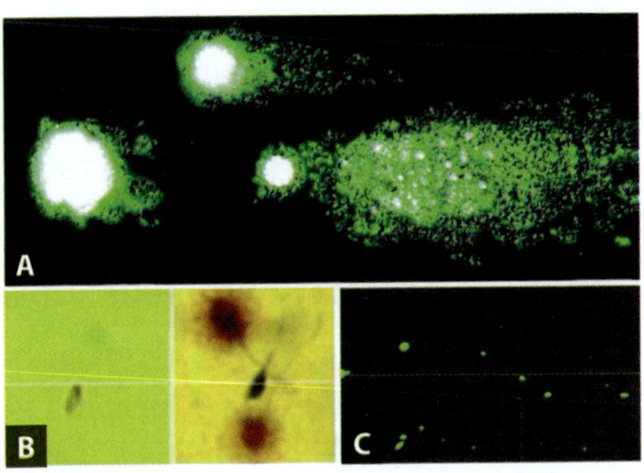

Figs. 3A to C: (A) Comet assay; (B) SCSA; (C) TUNEL assay. (SCSA: sperm chromatin structure assay; TUNEL: terminal deoxynucleotidyl transferase dUTP nick end labeling)

ART and there was an increase in SDF in approximately 50% of patients especially when higher centrifugation force, longer duration, and Percoll gradients were used leading to poor pregnancy rates.

MANAGEMENT OF HIGH SPERM DNA FRAGMENTATION

Lifestyle Modifications

- To quit smoking and alcohol consumption
- Regular exercise and weight reduction
- To wear loose garments
- Avoid high temperatures such as sauna baths and high-temperature workspaces.

Decrease DNA Damage

This can be accomplished by frequent ejaculation, especially around the time of ovulation. This reduces DNA damage by reducing the sperm transit time through the epididymis which reduces the exposure time to OS.

Short Ejaculatory Abstinence

Daily ejaculation for four consecutive days in patients with high SDF is a cost-effective method of reducing SDF without compromising other semen parameters.[9]

Oral Antioxidant Therapy

Antioxidants scavenge the excess free radicals and prevent oxidative damage to macromolecules. They are commonly used to maintain redox balance by scavenging ROS. Even though studies have shown a positive effect of antioxidant supplementation, there are no validated guidelines on antioxidant supplementation. The most commonly used antioxidants are zinc (400 mg), vitamin E up to 1,000 mg, and vitamin C up to 1,000 mg for 3–6 months. Even though antioxidants have been shown to improve the live birth rate, further research is needed to identify the ideal candidates and treatment regimens.[10] However, excess antioxidant supplementation may have a paradoxical effect on OS and SDF referred to as "reductive stress". So indiscriminate use of oral antioxidants in men should be avoided.

Control of Infections/Inflammation/Leukocytospermia

The incidence of infection varies from 2 to 18%. Sexually transmitted disease and prostatitis are associated with elevated ROS and leukocytospermia which can lead to elevated SDF. Antibiotic treatment has been effective in improving infection-elevated SDF. The drugs commonly used are macrolide, tetracycline, or quinolones.

Varicocelectomy

It is one of the correctable causes and proper selection of patients for varicocele ligation should be considered as pregnancy is observed in only 40–50% of patients undergoing varicocele ligation. Men with varicocele have significantly higher SDF, abnormal DNA packaging, and mitochondrial membrane potential. A review assessed the effect of varicocele ligation on SDF in >1,200 subjects. They observed a significant decrease in SDF following varicocele ligation during a follow-up of 3–12 months.[11]

Sperm Processing and Preparation

Certain laboratory conditions like prolonged incubation, centrifugation, cryopreservation, and use of different media can increase OS-mediated DNA damage and impact SDF. Conventional swim-up, density gradient, and advanced techniques such as magnetic activated cell sorting (MACS) can select sperms with low SDF. Intracytoplasmic morphologically selected sperm injection (IMSI) uses high magnification to select morphologically normal sperms as the presence of vacuoles in the nuclear region is associated with high SDF. Other techniques include physiological intracytoplasmic sperm injection (PICSI) and microfluidic devices that can select sperms with less SDF.

Use of Testicular Sperm for Intracytoplasmic Sperm Injection

Testicular sperms have been shown to have lower SDF than ejaculated sperms with better ICSI outcomes.[12] However, there is a risk of anesthesia and surgical complications in addition to the possible concern of a higher aneuploidy rate in testicular sperms. So, the use of testicular sperms in nonazoospermic patients is still debatable.

EFFECT OF SPERM DNA FRAGMENTATION ON OUTCOMES

Natural Conception

The integrity of sperm DNA plays a crucial role in the process of fertilization, early embryo development, and hence the chances of natural conception. It is shown that high SDF is associated with low cleavage rates and arrest of embryonic development.[13] In a meta-analysis revealed that high SDF by SCSA test was associated with failure to achieve natural pregnancy with an odd's ratio of 7.01 [95% confidence interval (CI): 3.68–13.36].[14]

Intrauterine Insemination

Chen et al. (2019) analyzed 10 studies and found that high SDF was associated with significantly lower pregnancy [relative risk (RR) = 0.34 95% CI: 0.22–0.52; p <0.001], delivery rates (RR: 0.14, 95% CI: 0.04–0.56; p <0.001)] but this is questioned by some of the studies as the positive predictive value of these tests are low.[15]

ASSISTED REPRODUCTIVE TECHNOLOGY (FLOWCHART 1)

Studies on the predictive role of SDF on ART are contradictory. This can be attributed to the heterogeneity of studies, different SDF testing, and female factors. Various meta-analyses have reported lower pregnancy rates with conventional in vitro fertilization (IVF) with or between 0.68 and 1.7. However, many studies have not found any association between ICSI and SDF except a study by Simon et al. which has reported significantly lower pregnancy rates with high SDF with ICSI.[16]

In a meta-analysis, the live birth rate was found to be significantly lower in men with high SDF following both IVF and ICSI with a combined or of 1.17 (95% CI: 1.07–1.28; $p = 0.0005$).[17] Similarly high SDF is associated with a greater risk of miscarriage after ART with OR between 2.28 and 2.48. However, contradictory results have been shown in some of the studies even though

Flowchart 1: Clinical algorithm to elucidate the applications of SDF testing in clinical practice.[4]

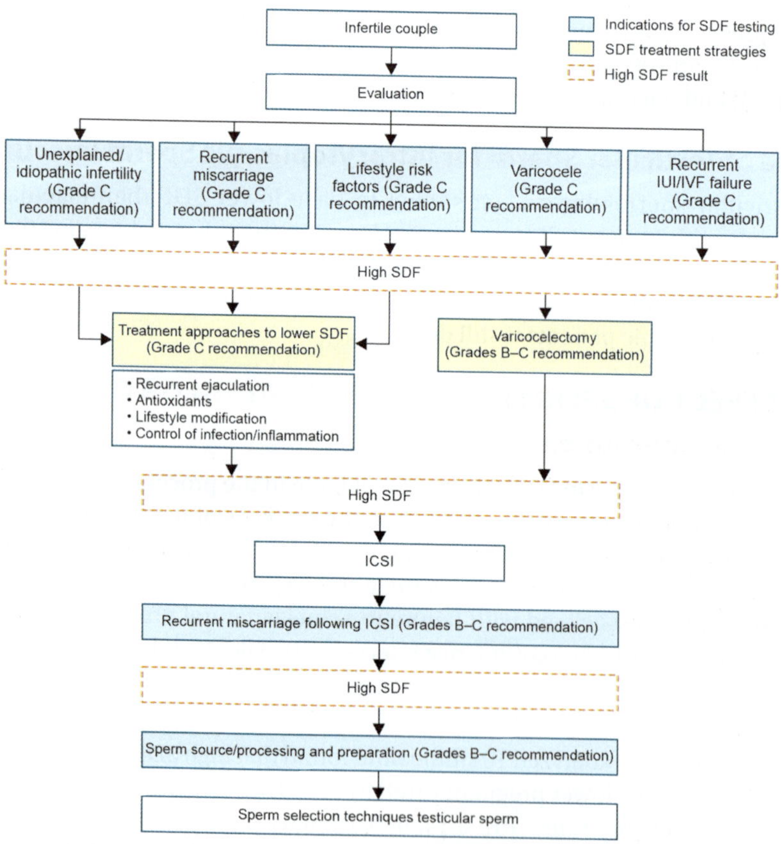

(ICSI: intracytoplasmic sperm injection; SDF: sperm deoxyribonucleic acid fragmentation)

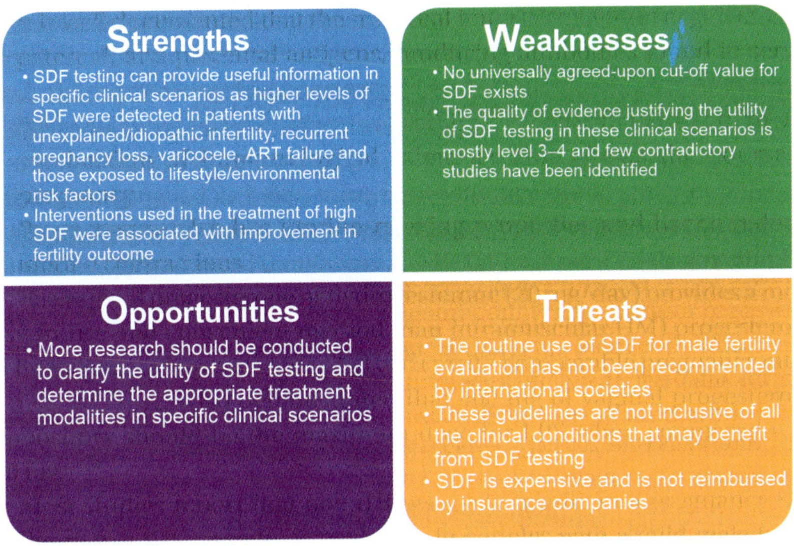

Fig. 4: SWOT analysis on the clinical utility of SDF.[4] (SWOT: strengths, weaknesses, opportunities, and threats; SDF: sperm deoxyribonucleic acid fragmentation)

tests had good sensitivity but poor specificity. It is shown that based on the receiver-operating characteristic (ROC) curve, TUNEL and Comet assay had fair predictive performance, and poor predictive power was noted with SCSA and SCD assays. A SWOT (strengths, weaknesses, opportunities, and threats) analysis is presented in **Figure 4**.

CONCLUSION

- SDF influences fertilization, embryo development, infertility treatment, and pregnancy outcome.
- There are several assay methods to assess SDF. The most commonly used tests are TUNEL assay, Comet assay, SCD, and SCSA.
- SDF testing is beneficial in patients with unexplained infertility, varicocele, and men with lifestyle risk factors, such as obesity, smoking, alcoholic, cancer, diabetes, and environmental hazards.
- High SDF can be treated with lifestyle modification, varicocelectomy in indicated cases, antioxidant therapy, and sperm selection techniques.

REFERENCES

1. Thonneau P, Marchand S, Tallec A, Ferial ML, Ducot B, Lansac J, et al. Incidence and main causes of infertility in a resident population (1,850,000) of three French regions (1988–1989). Hum Reprod. 1991;6(6):811-6.
2. Agarwal A, Said TM. Role of sperm chromatin abnormalities and DNA damage in male infertility. Hum Reprod Update. 2003;9(4):331-45.

3. Sharma RK, Sabanegh E, Mahfouz R, Gupta S, Thiyagarajan A, Agarwal A. TUNEL as a test for sperm DNA damage in the evaluation of male infertility. Urology. 2010;76(6):1380-6.
4. Agarwal A, Majzoub A, Baskaran S, Panner Selvam MK, Cho CL, Henkel R, et al. Sperm DNA Fragmentation: A New Guideline for Clinicians. World J Mens Health. 2020;38(4):412-71.
5. Wang YJ, Zhang RQ, Lin YJ, Zhang RG, Zhang WL. Relationship between varicocele and sperm DNA damage and the effect of varicocele repair: a meta-analysis. Reprod Biomed Online. 2012;25(3):307-14.
6. Agarwal A, Majzoub A, Esteves SC, Ko E, Ramasamy R, Zini A. Clinical utility of sperm DNA fragmentation testing: practice recommendations based on clinical scenarios. Transl Androl Urol. 2017;6(Suppl 4):S720-33.
7. De Iuliis GN, Newey RJ, King BV, Aitken RJ. Mobile phone radiation induces reactive oxygen species production and DNA damage in human spermatozoa in vitro. PLoS One. 2009;4(7):e6446.
8. Esteves SC, Sánchez-Martín F, Sánchez-Martín P, Schneider DT, Gosálvez J. Comparison of reproductive outcome in oligozoospermic men with high sperm DNA fragmentation undergoing intracytoplasmic sperm injection with ejaculated and testicular sperm. Fertil Steril. 2015;104(6):1398-405.
9. Kaur B, Prakash V, Malik S, Bhatia V, Grover A, Gupta D. Role of daily ejaculation for four consecutive days in improving sperm DNA fragmentation index. Fertil Sci Res. 2020;7(1):85-91.
10. Smits RM, Mackenzie-Proctor R, Yazdani A, Stankiewicz MT, Jordan V, Showell MG. Antioxidants for male subfertility. Cochrane Database Syst Rev. 2019;3:CD0074119.
11. Roque M, Esteves SC. Effect of varicocele repair on sperm DNA fragmentation: a review. Int Urol Nephrol. 2018;50(4):583-603.
12. Bradley CK, McArthur SJ, Gee AJ, Weiss KA, Schmidt U, Toogood L. Intervention improves assisted conception intracytoplasmic sperm injection outcomes for patients with high levels of sperm DNA fragmentation: a retrospective analysis. Andrology. 2016;4(5):903-10.
13. Ruvolo G, Fattouh RR, Bosco L, Brucculeri AM, Cittadini E. New molecular markers for the evaluation of gamete quality. J Assist Reprod Genet. 2013; 30(2):207-12.
14. Zini A, Boman JM, Belzile E, Ciampi A. Sperm DNA damage is associated with an increased risk of pregnancy loss after IVF and ICSI: systematic review and meta-analysis. Hum Reprod. 2008;23(12):2663-8.
15. Chen Q, Zhao JY, Xue X, Zhu GX. The association between sperm DNA fragmentation and reproductive outcomes following intrauterine insemination, a meta analysis. Reprod Toxicol. 2019;86:50-5.
16. Simon L, Zini A, Dyachenko A, Ciampi A, Carrell DT. A systematic review and meta-analysis to determine the effect of sperm DNA damage on in vitro fertilization and intracytoplasmic sperm injection outcome. Asian J Androl. 2017;19(1):80-90.
17. Osman A, Alsomait H, Seshadri S, El-Toukhy T, Khalaf Y. The effect of sperm DNA fragmentation on live birth rate after IVF or ICSI: a systematic review and meta-analysis. Reprod Biomed Online. 2015;30(2):120-7.

CHAPTER 8

Dealing with Urological Injuries

HP Pattnaik, Pratik Tambe

INTRODUCTION

Urological injuries are a common complication in gynecological surgery. These injuries can be caused by various factors including surgical technique, variations in patient anatomy, and preexisting medical conditions. Lower urinary tract injuries may occur during gynecological surgery due to the close proximity of pelvic organs and vary by procedure, surgical indication, and route or approach. Prevention of such injuries should be a primary goal during any gynecological surgery. They may be more common during difficult procedures and with surgeons who have less experience.

Immediate recognition and primary management of injuries are ideal, although delayed postoperative diagnoses may happen in certain cases. Surgical management is based on the size and location of an injury and should be performed by an experienced surgeon with thorough knowledge of pelvic anatomy, surgical technique, and postoperative management. Urological injuries can have significant implications for patient outcomes including prolonged hospital stays, increased morbidity and mortality, and decreased quality of life.[1]

TYPES OF UROLOGICAL INJURIES DURING GYNECOLOGICAL SURGERY

Urological injuries in gynecological surgery can involve the bladder, urethra, ureters, and rarely, the kidneys. The most common urological injuries are bladder injuries, which occur in up to 1% of all gynecological surgeries. Ureteric injuries are less common, occurring in 0.5–1% of surgeries but are most dreaded, while urethral injuries are even rarer with an incidence of <0.1%.

Bladder Injury

Bladder injury can occur during a variety of gynecological procedures, including hysterectomy, myomectomy, and pelvic floor repair. These injuries can range from minor bladder wall lacerations to full-thickness injuries that extend into the peritoneal cavity. Bladder injuries can lead to urine leakage, infection, and even urosepsis.

Ureteric Injury

Ureteric injury can occur during surgeries that involve manipulation of the pelvic organs such as hysterectomy, pelvic lymph node dissection, and ovarian cystectomy. These injuries can range from partial or complete transection of the ureter to avulsion of the ureter from its insertion into the bladder. Ureteric injuries can lead to urinary tract obstruction, hydronephrosis, and renal failure.

Urethral Injury

Urethral injury is rare during gynecological surgery but can occur during procedures that involve the anterior vaginal wall such as anterior colporrhaphy or sling surgery. Urethral injuries can range from minor tears to complete transection of the urethra. Urethral injuries can lead to urinary incontinence, urethral stricture, and urinary tract infections.

RISK FACTORS FOR UROLOGICAL INJURIES

Several risk factors can increase the likelihood of urological injuries in gynecological surgery. These risk factors include:

- Previous pelvic surgery or radiation therapy, which can lead to adhesions and scarring that make surgical dissection more difficult.
- Obesity, which can increase the difficulty of surgical dissection and increase the risk of injury to adjacent organs.
- Endometriosis, which can lead to distortion and fixation of pelvic organs, making surgical dissection more difficult.
- Large fibroids or ovarian cysts, which can make surgical dissection more difficult and increase the risk of injury to adjacent organs.
- Pelvic organs prolapse, which can increase the risk of urethral injury during anterior vaginal wall surgery.

PREVENTION AND MANAGEMENT OF UROLOGICAL INJURIES

Prevention and management of urological injuries in gynecological surgery require a multidisciplinary approach involving the surgeon, anesthetist, urologist, and experienced nursing team. The following strategies can help prevent urological injuries:

- Preoperative assessment of urinary tract anatomy, including imaging studies, such as cystoscopy, ureteroscopy, and magnetic resonance imaging (MRI).
- Intraoperative identification and protection of the ureters and bladder during surgical dissection, using techniques, such as bladder dissection with a Foley catheter in place, intraoperative cystoscopy, and ureteric stenting.
- Use of appropriate surgical techniques and instruments, such as laparoscopic or robotic surgery, to minimize the risk of injury to adjacent organs.

- Adequate tissue mobilization and visualization during surgery to minimize the risk of accidental injury to adjacent organs.

If a urological injury does occur during gynecological surgery, prompt recognition and management are essential. The following steps can help manage urological injuries:

- Immediate cessation of surgery and assessment of the extent and location of the injury.
- Referral to a urologist or general surgeon at the earliest.
- Placement of a ureteric stent or nephrostomy tube to relieve obstruction and prevent further renal damage.
- Repair of the injury, either by primary closure or by diversion of urine flow if necessary.
- Close monitoring of the patient for signs of infection, urinary leakage, or renal dysfunction.

Injuries during Cesarean Section

A team from Israel has reported on their 14-year-long experience of urological injuries during Caesarean section. A total of 17,794 cesarean deliveries (17.5%) were performed. 14 cases of bladder injury (0.08%) and 11 cases of ureteric injury (0.06%) were identified. All bladder injuries were diagnosed and repaired intraoperatively. Six (55%) cases of ureteric injury were diagnosed in the postoperative period and three of these required further surgery for definitive treatment. None of the patients suffered long-term adverse effects.

Most bladder injuries occurred in women with previous cesarean delivery in the presence of abdominal adhesions. In contrast, most ureteric injuries occurred in women with emergency Cesarean delivery during the second stage of labor and were accompanied by an extension of the uterine incision. All women had normal kidney function in follow-up and did not suffer from long-term sequelae.[2]

Vaginal Birth after Cesarean Section

Urological injuries have been reported in women undergoing trials of labor and vaginal birth after cesarean section (VBAC). Uterine rupture is associated with an elevated risk of bladder and ureteric injury. The incidence of bladder injury varies between 8 and 15% in published literature, with the highest being after a failed trial of VBAC. The clinical picture is diverse and includes hematuria (most frequently), severe lower abdominal pain, vaginal bleeding, palpation of fetal parts, cessation of uterine contractions, nonreassuring fetal heart tracing, and maternal shock. Other rare signs include vernixuria, oligoanuria, and the presence of meconium in urine.[3-5]

Iatrogenic Ureteric Injury

Most iatrogenic ureteric injuries are in the form of incomplete transection, but perforation (partial or complete), ligation, or complete transection can also occur. One review reported that 38% of ureteral injuries are initially missing. Long-term complications of missed ureteral injuries include urinoma, ileus, periureteral abscess, sepsis, ureteral fistula, or ureteral stricture.[6]

The density of intra-abdominal adhesions after cesarean births is increasing and is related to the number of previous cesareans. The adhesion rates vary from 12 to 46% in patients with two cesarean sections to 26–75% in those with three cesarean sections. One theory for bladder-ureteric injuries suggests that there may be a rupture of dense adhesions between the bladder and uterus caused by high peritonization during the previous cesarean section, by an irregular apposition of the edges in multiple scars of the uterus or the presence of associated endometriotic lesions.[7,8]

Management for ureteric injuries is discussed in **Flowchart 1**.

Urogenital Fistulas

Long-term complications stemming from urinary tract injuries include urogenital fistulas. Obstetric fistulas are rare in modern medicine as

Flowchart 1: Management algorithm for ureteric injuries.[9]

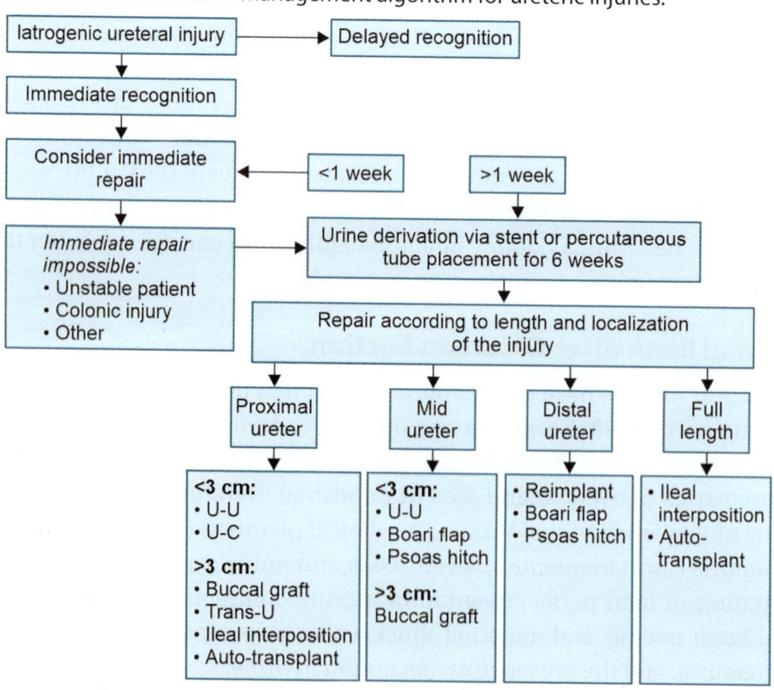

most cases are identified after performing an instrumental delivery. Most vesicouterine and vesicovaginal fistulas occur after cesarean section and uterine rupture. Intraoperative recognition aids in successful primary repair.

Late presentations present a challenge as these may become symptomatic weeks to months after the primary surgery. These are usually the result of injury by grasping, crushing, kinking, or cauterization. The lack of blood supply leads to avascular necrosis and a late presentation in these patients. Multidisciplinary care and careful identification of the site of fistula with appropriate corrective surgery is necessary.[10]

Repair of Bladder Injuries

Bladder injuries whether intraperitoneal or extraperitoneal are repaired using a two-layer technique; the first layer is a running 3-0 absorbable suture. The second layer is a running 2-0 or 3-0 absorbable suture. An indwelling urethral catheter drainage is recommended for 3 weeks. Prolonged bladder catheterization exposes the patient to an increased risk of urinary tract infection and regular bladder washes are necessary in the postoperative period. Administration of methylene blue dye can be helpful in assessing the integrity of the lower urinary tract. A cystogram may be performed before catheter removal to evaluate healing.

The bladder is re-epithelialized in 3–4 days and regains its normal function after 21 days; bladder training is required in the postoperative period. Good antibiotic coverage is essential. Supratrigonal injuries are usually repaired with excellent results if they are recognized intraoperatively. However, injuries to the trigone or below the trigone may involve the ureters or urethra and are significantly more challenging to repair than injuries at the level of the bladder dome or above the trigone. Exposure and closure in this area is difficult and may require ureteric stenting additionally.[11]

INJURIES DURING LAPAROSCOPIC AND ROBOTIC SURGERY

A systematic review published in 2021 found the overall urinary tract injury rate for laparoscopic hysterectomy was 0.73%. The bladder injury rate ranged from 0.05 to 0.66% across procedure types and the ureteric injury rate ranged from 0.02 to 0.4%. In contrast to earlier publications that cited unacceptably high urinary tract injury rates, laparoscopic hysterectomy appears to be safe regarding injuries to the bladder and ureter.[12]

Data published from Detroit, Michigan showed a total of 3,114 hysterectomies, of which 1,088 were robotic, 782 laparoscopic, 304 vaginal, and 940 abdominal hysterectomies. A total of 27 injuries were confirmed (seven during laparoscopic hysterectomy, 10 during robotic hysterectomy, one during vaginal hysterectomy, and nine during abdominal hysterectomy). The overall rate of urological injury was 0.87% with a 0.55% risk of bladder injury and a 0.32% risk of injury to the ureter.

When the route of hysterectomy was taken into account, the risk of urological injury was 0.92% for robotic hysterectomy, 0.90% for laparoscopic hysterectomy, 0.33% for vaginal hysterectomy and 0.96% for open hysterectomy. The mean body mass index (BMI) for all patients was 32.7 kg/m^2; injured patients had a mean BMI of 34.6 kg/m^2, and noninjured patients had a mean BMI of 32.0 kg/m^2 ($p = 0.10$). They concluded that the rates of urologic injury with robotic hysterectomy are similar to those of laparoscopic hysterectomy. BMI was not significantly different in patients who had urological injuries.[13]

LARGEST PUBLISHED SYSTEMATIC REVIEW

The findings of a large systematic review published in 2023 included 96 eligible studies and 1,741,894 women. Amongst women undergoing cesarean section, weighted pooled rates of bladder or ureteric injury per 100,000 procedures were 267 or nine events, respectively.

Injury rates during hysterectomy varied by approach and pathological condition. Weighted pooled mean rates for bladder injury were 212–997 events per 100,000 procedures for all approaches (open, vaginal, laparoscopic, laparoscopically assisted vaginal, and robot-assisted) and all pathological conditions (benign, malignant, and any), except for open peripartum hysterectomy (6,279 events) and laparoscopic hysterectomy for malignancy (1,553 events).

Similarly, weighted pooled mean rates for ureteric injury were 9–577 events per 100,000 procedures for all hysterectomy approaches and pathologies, except for open peripartum hysterectomy (666 events) and laparoscopic hysterectomy for malignancy (814 events). Surgeon inexperience was the prime risk factor for injury and improved anatomical knowledge was the leading preventative strategy.[14]

CONCLUSION

Urological injuries are a common complication in gynecological surgery, with bladder injuries being the most common and urethral injuries being the least common. Several risk factors can increase the likelihood of urological injuries including previous pelvic surgery or radiation therapy, obesity, endometriosis, large fibroids or ovarian cysts, and pelvic organ prolapse.

Prevention and management of urological injuries require a multidisciplinary approach involving the surgeon, anesthetist, urologist, and a well-experienced nursing team. Adequate tissue mobilization and visualization during surgery, use of appropriate surgical techniques and instruments, and intraoperative identification and protection of the ureters and bladder can help prevent urological injuries. If a urological injury does occur, prompt recognition and management are essential to minimize morbidity and mortality and ensure a good outcome.

REFERENCES

1. Patel UJ, Heisler CA. Urinary tract injury during gynecologic surgery: prevention, recognition, and management. Obstet Gynecol Clin North Am. 2021;48(3):535-56.
2. Safrai M, Stern S, Gofrit ON, Hidas G, Kabiri D. Urinary tract injuries during cesarean delivery: long-term outcome and management. J Matern Fetal Neonatal Med. 2022;35(18):3547-54.
3. Varlas VN, Rhazi Y, Bors RG, Penes O, Radavoi D. The urological complications of vaginal birth after cesarean (VBAC): a literature review. J Med Life. 2021;14(4):443-7.
4. Tähtinen RM, Cartwright R, Tsui JF, Aaltonen RL, Aoki Y, Cárdenas JL, et al. Long term impact of mode of delivery on stress urinary incontinence and urgency urinary incontinence: a systematic review and meta-analysis. Eur Urol. 2016;70(1):148-58.
5. Fishel Bartal M, Sibai BM, Ilan H, Fried M, Rahav R, Alexandroni H, et al. Trial of labor after cesarean (TOLAC) in women with premature rupture of membranes. J Matern Fetal Neonatal Med. 2020;33(17):2976-82.
6. Phillips B, Holzmer S, Turco L, Mirzaie M, Mause E, Mause A, et al. Trauma to the bladder and ureter: a review of diagnosis, management, and prognosis. Eur J Trauma Emerg Surg. 2017;43(6):763-73.
7. Uyanikoglu H, Karahan MA, Turp AB, Agar M, Tasduzen ME, Sak S, et al. Are multiple repeated cesarean sections really as safe? J Matern Fetal Neonatal Med. 2017;30(4):482-85.
8. Filip L, Duică F, Prădatu A, Crețoiu D, Suciu N, Crețoiu SM, et al. Endometriosis associated infertility: a critical review and analysis on etiopathogenesis and therapeutic approaches. Medicina (Kaunas). 2020;56(9):460.
9. Smith AP, Bazinet A, Liberman D. Iatrogenic ureteral injury after gynecological surgery. Can Urol Assoc J. 2019;13(6 Suppl4):S51-5.
10. Gilmour DT, Vallis TM, Lee W, Colford D, Reardon E. Minimizing the urological and psychological morbidity of urinary tract fistulae from VBAC. J Obstet Gynaecol Can. 2006;28(2):132-5.
11. Tarney CM. Bladder injury during cesarean delivery. Curr Womens Health Rev. 2013;9(2):70-6.
12. Adelman MR, Bardsley TR, Sharp HT. Urinary tract injuries in laparoscopic hysterectomy: a systematic review. J Minim Invasive Gynecol. 2014;21(4):558-66.
13. Petersen SS, Doe S, Rubinfeld I, Davydova Y, Buekers T, Sangha R. Rate of urologic injury with robotic hysterectomy. J Minim Invasive Gynecol. 2018;25(5):867-71.
14. Wei G, Harley F, O'Callaghan M, Adshead J, Hennessey D, Kinnear N. Systematic review of urological injury during caesarean section and hysterectomy. Int Urogynecol J. 2023;34(2):371-89.

CHAPTER 9

Modern Methodology in Screening for Breast Cancer

Karishma Kirti, Nita S Nair, Sridevi Murali-Nanavati

INTRODUCTION

Breast cancer is the most common cancer among women worldwide. In 2018, India reported 162,468 new cases, making it the leading cancer in women (27.7%) and the cause of 11.1% of all cancer deaths that year.[1] The incidence of breast cancer is rising with a significant urban-to-rural divide.[2]

Screening is defined as the identification of an unrecognized disease in an apparently healthy, asymptomatic population by means of tests, examinations, or other procedures that can be applied rapidly and easily to the target population **(Box 1)**.

The accuracy of a screening test hinges on its capability to differentiate between the presence of disease and its absence. Concerns regarding biases in screening include lead time, length time, and selection bias **(Table 1)** **(Figs. 1A and B)**. Overdiagnosis is a concerning outcome of screening, causing anxiety and straining healthcare systems.

SCREENING IN BREAST CANCER

Over the years, screening for breast cancer has become synonymous with the use of mammography (MMG) alone. However, the role of physical examination or clinical breast examination (CBE) by trained healthcare professionals needs to be given due consideration. Ideally, a screening tool for breast cancer should aim to reduce mortality from both breast cancer and all-cause mortality, maintain a low false positive rate, and be inexpensive.

BOX 1: Principles of screening.

The effectiveness of any screening is measured by various means.

Disease requirements:

- Disease must be serious in nature with significant rates of morbidity and/or mortality
- Effective treatment should be available
- Natural history should be well understood to identify the window of opportunity for early detection and effective treatment or possibly a cure
- Disease must not be too rare

Screening test requirements:

- Easy and inexpensive
- Safe and acceptable to individuals as well as physicians
- Reproducible
- Level of accuracy should be adequate

Healthcare system requirements: Accessible cancer care is essential for positive cases

TABLE 1: Biases associated with screening.

Lead time bias	Increased survival is a function of the time gained before the point at which the disease would have become evident in the absence of screening although the time of death remains the same **(Fig. 1A)**
Length time bias	The tendency to detect slow-growing tumors as more aggressive tumors are likely to presents interval cancers **(Fig. 1B)**
Selection bias	It is the tendency for individuals who are health conscious to participate in screening trials
Overdiagnosis bias	Diagnosis of a disease that could have potentially not been diagnosed throughout life with death due to another cause eventually

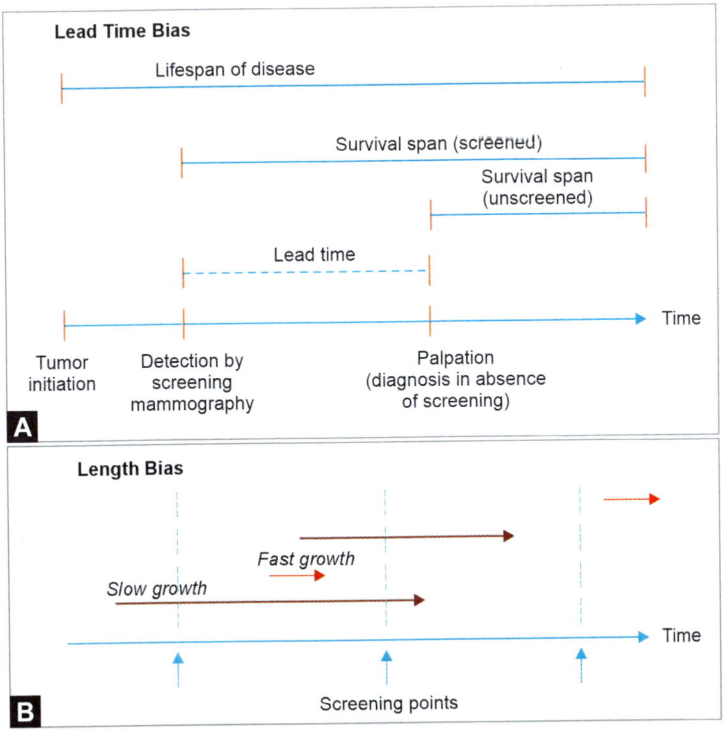

Figs. 1A and B: (A) Lead time bias; (B) Length bias.

AVAILABLE MODALITIES FOR SCREENING

- Breast self-examination (BSE)
- CBE
- Screening by imaging—mammogram
- Ultrasound/magnetic resonance imaging (MRI)

Breast Self-Examination

Due to its simplicity and affordability, BSE appears to be the most suitable approach for early breast cancer screening. Nonetheless, there is a lack of studies demonstrating its impact on mortality reduction. Two landmark randomized controlled trials have assessed the efficacy of BSE as a screening method.

1. *Shanghai trial:*[3] In this trial, a total of 266,064 factory workers in Shanghai participated. Women were randomly assigned to either the BSE instruction group or the non-instruction group. Tumor size, stage, and cumulative breast cancer mortality rates did not exhibit significant differences between the two groups. The study concluded that providing intensive instruction in BSE does not lead to a reduction in breast cancer mortality rates; however, it did reveal an increase in the detection of smaller benign breast lumps.
2. *Russian trial:*[4] This study of 122,471 women from St Petersburg, were randomly assigned to either BSE or not. Results showed no difference in mortality, but the BSE group had a slightly higher 15-year survival rate (53.2% vs. 45.8%, $p = 0.051$). The indications for biopsy were more than double in the experimental arm (7.5% vs. 3.5%, $p < 0.01$).

A meta-analysis by Hackshaw et al.,[5] which encompassed these two randomized controlled trials (RCTs) along with 20 observational studies, similarly concluded that BSE does not effectively reduce breast cancer mortality. The success of BSE depends on the subject's motivation and her recognition of breast cancer as a real threat to her. Studies have shown poor participation rates in breast teaching classes and low compliance with monthly breast examinations. Nevertheless, it does contribute to greater awareness about breast cancer and overall breast health.

Clinical Breast Examination

The role of MMG as a screening tool has faced criticism over the years. It has shown low sensitivity in premenopausal women, sparking debates about its efficacy as a screening tool. However, in women above 50 years of age, MMG either alone or combined with CBE has shown a reduction in cause-specific mortality. Unfortunately, it has also resulted in approximately 25% overdiagnosis after 25 years of follow-up.[6] Transitioning to CBE may reduce the detection of indolent invasive as well as noninvasive cancers and potentially reduce overdiagnosis. There are three randomized controlled trials that directly evaluate the role of CBE in breast cancer.

1. *The Philippines study:*[7] In 1995, Pisani et al. conducted a randomized trial involving women aged 35–64 years. They were either assigned to five annual clinical examinations of the breasts (carried out by trained nurses/midwives) versus not. The first round of examination round involved 151,168 women who were also trained in BSE techniques and provided with a leaflet

in the local language explaining the purpose and methodology of BSE. Due to poor compliance with follow-up for screen-positive women, even with home visits, the active intervention was discontinued after completing the first screening round in December 1997.

2. *The Trivandrum study:*[8] Sankarnarayanan et al., initiated a study in the Trivandrum district in 2006 wherein they randomized 115,652 healthy women, aged 30–69 years to either intervention (CBE) or control (no screening). The percentage of early-stage (stage IIA or lower) breast cancers detected in the intervention vs. control groups was 43.8% versus 25.4% ($p = 0.023$), while advanced-stage (stage IIB or higher) breast cancers detected were 45.0% versus 68.3% ($p = 0.005$). Thus, suggesting that there was a downstaging of cancers noted in the CBE arm.
3. *The Mumbai study:*[9] A 20-year prospective, cluster-randomized controlled trial initiated in 1998 by Mittra et al., involved 151,538 women aged 35–64 years with no prior breast cancer history. The study compared two groups: (1) The intervention group (n = 75,360 received CBE by healthcare workers and cancer awareness every 2 years, followed by five rounds of active surveillance every 2 years) and (2) the control group (n = 76,178 received one round of cancer awareness followed by eight rounds of active surveillance every 2 years). The results show that the intervention group experienced a significant downstaging of breast cancer at diagnosis, with a nonsignificant 15% reduction in overall breast cancer mortality. Notably, there was a substantial and significant 30% reduction in mortality among women aged 50 years and older. No significant change in mortality was seen in women under 50 years of age. The intervention group also showed a 5% decrease in all-cause mortality, though this was not statistically significant. These findings underscore the potential value of CBE for breast cancer screening in low- and middle-income countries **(Tables 2 and 3)**.

The efficacy of randomized controlled studies for combined modality breast cancer screening (MMG and CBE) is highlighted in **Table 4**.

TABLE 2: Staging at diagnosis (breast-screening arm).

Monitoring rounds	*Early stage (0 + I + II)*	*Late stage (III + IV)*	*Staging not available*	*Total*
One	21 (70.00%)	9 (30.00%)	2	32
Interval cancers	17 (73.91%)	6 (26.09%)	4	27
Two	15 (68.18%)	7 (31.82%)	2	24
Interval cancers	13 (92.86%)	1 (7.14%)	3	17
Three	12 (57.14%)	9 (42.86%)	4	25

TABLE 3: Staging of asymptomatic referrals at diagnosis (breast-control arm).

Monitoring rounds	*Early stage (0 + I + II)*	*Late stage (III+ IV)*	*Staging not available*	*Total*
One	2 (66.67%)	1 (33.33%)	0	3
Two	18 (54.55%)	15 (45.45%)	6	39
Three	18 (46.15%)	21 (53.85%)	6	45

TABLE 4: Efficacy of randomized controlled studies for combined modality breast cancer screening (MMG and CBE).

Study	*Cancers detected in the screened population*	*Interval cancers*	*CBE*		*Downstaging*	
			Sensitivity	*Specificity*	*Screened*	*Control*
Mumbai study	73	37	57.44%	91.99%	*Early:* 78 *Advanced:* 38	*Early:* 32 *Advanced:* 37
Philippines study	68	NA	53.2%	100%	17% more advanced cases in control group	
Trivandrum Study	80	28	54.1%	94%	*Early:* 43.8 *Advanced:* 45.0	*Early:* 25.4 *Advanced:* 68.3

IMAGING MODALITIES

Mammography

Numerous RCTs have investigated the efficacy of screening MMG in breast cancer detection **(Table 5)**.

- *The Health Insurance Plan (HIP) study*[10] was the pioneering RCT which was designed to demonstrate the role of screening in mortality reduction in breast cancer, using MMG and CBE (by trained surgeons). It involved 6,200 women aged 40–64 years. After 18 years, the results showed a relative risk (RR) for breast cancer mortality of 0.77 (0.52–1.13) for women aged 40–49 years, 0.79 (0.58–1.08) for women aged 50–64 years and an overall RR of 0.78 (0.61–1.00).
- *The Edinburgh randomized trial* of breast cancer screening[11] enrolled 44,288 women aged 45–64 years from 1978 to 81. Among them, 22,944 were randomized to receive 7 years of screening, while the rest served as controls. After 10 years, breast cancer mortality was 14–21% lower in the study group although this difference did not reach statistical significance.

TABLE 5: Screening details of the randomized trials of breast cancer screening using mammography.

Study	*Year*	*Age at entry*	*Numbers screened*		*Screening interval and rounds of screening 5 rounds MMG + CBE versus CBE/not and no of rounds of screening*	*Available follow-up*
			Screened	*Control*		
HIP	1963–1969	40–64 years	31,000	31,000	Annual MMG + CBE vs not 3 rounds	18 years
Edinburgh	1978–1991	45–64 years	22,944	21,344	2 yearly MMG + annual CBE (7 rounds)	10 years
CNBSS I	1980	40–49 years	44,925	44,910	Annual MMG + CBE + BSE versus one-time CBE + BSE at initial evaluation	25 years
CNBSS II	1980	50–59 years			Annual MMG + CBE + BSE versus annual CBE + BSE	25 years
UK Age Trial	1990–1997	39–41 years	53,883	106,953	Annual MMG	22.8 years
Malmö I	1976–1978	45–70 years	21,088	21,195	MMG every 18–24 months (five rounds)	30 years
Malmö II	1978–1990	43–49 years	9,587	8,199	MMG every 18–24 months	22 years
Swedish Two-County Trial	1977–1979	40–74 years	77,080	55,985	40–49 years—MMG every 2 years 50–74 years—MMG every 3 years	29 years
Stockholm Trial	1981–1985	40–64 years	40,318	20,000	MMG every 2 years (two rounds)	25 years
Göteborg Trial	1982–1991	39–59 years	21,650	29,961	MMG every 18 months (five rounds)	25 years

(BSE: breast self-examination; CBE: clinical breast examination; MMG: mammography)

- *Canadian National Breast Screening Study I and II:*[12] This is the sole randomized study that addresses the role of MMG alongside CBE. Nearly 90,000 women were randomized in the CNBSS studies.
  - *CNBSS 1* randomized 50,489 women aged 40–49 years old to MMG + CBE versus standard healthcare. At the end of a 16-year follow-up, there was no significant difference in BC mortality between the two groups.
  - *CNBSS II* included women aged 50–59 years and randomized them to annual MMG + CBE + BSE to annual CBE + BSE alone to assess the impact of adding MMG.

  MMG + CBE + BSE detected more node-negative and small breast cancers than screening with CBE + BSE alone, but this had no impact on breast cancer mortality. The risk of a false positive result was 49.1% [95% confidence interval (CI) 40.3–64.1] after 10 MMGs and 22.3 % (95% CI 19.2–27.5) after 10 CBEs.[13]

  At 25 years of follow-up,[13] among the 666 cancers detected in the MMG arm during the screening period, 454 cancers detected in the MMG arm and 524 in the control arm were palpable tumors. One overdiagnosed breast cancer was identified for every 424 women who received MMG screening. Overall, 1,005 women died from breast cancer during the 25-year follow-up period (1.1%). The 25-year cumulative mortality from all causes of death and breast cancer-specific mortality was similar between the MMG and control arms (1.02, 0.98–1.06; $p = 0.28$) and (0.99, 0.88–1.12; $p = 0.87$), respectively.
- *UK age trial:*[14] 160,921 women aged 39–41 years were randomly assigned in a 1:2 ratio to either an intervention group receiving annual MMG or a control group receiving standard medical care Over a median follow-up of 22.8 years, there was a significant 25% reduction in breast cancer mortality at 10 years, with 83 breast cancer deaths in the intervention group compared to 219 in the control group (RR: 0.75, 95% CI: 0.58–0.97, $p = 0.029$). However, no significant reduction was observed beyond 10 years of follow-up, with 126 deaths versus 255 deaths (RR: 0.98, 95% CI: 0.79–1.22, $p = 0.86$). This suggests that starting yearly MMG before age 50 years, specifically at ages 40 or 41 years, could potentially reduce breast cancer mortality, with a constant absolute reduction over time.
- *The Malmö trial:*[15] This study randomized birth year cohorts into screening versus no screening. Overall, women aged 55 years and older in the study group had a 20% reduction in breast cancer mortality [35 vs. 44; RR: 0.79 (0.51–1.24)]. A more recent related study[16] assessed the rate of overdiagnosis in the screening group at the end of 15 years and found it to be 10% in the 55–69 year age group.
- *Swedish Two-County trial:*[17] Involving 133,065 women aged 40–74 years in two Swedish counties (Dalarna and Östergötland), this trial randomized

them into a group invited to mammographic screening and a control group receiving usual care. There was a significant reduction in breast cancer mortality in women invited to screening according to both local endpoint committee data (RR = 0.69; 95% CI: 0.56–0.84; p <0.0001) and consensus data (RR = 0.73; 95% CI: 0.59–0.89; p = 0.002). At 29 years of follow-up, the number of women needed to undergo screening for 7 years to prevent one breast cancer death was 414 according to local data, and 519 according to consensus data.

- *Stockholm mammographic screening trial:*[18] 40,318 women aged 40–64 years were randomized for single view MMG for two screening rounds versus no intervention. Overall, after a mean follow-up of 11.2 years, a nonsignificant mortality reduction of 26% was seen. In women aged 40–49 years, there was no effect on mortality was found, while in the 50–64 year age group a significant 38% reduction in mortality was observed.
- *Göteborg breast screening trial:*[19] This trial randomized 51,611 women aged 39–49 years to MMG screening every 18 months. They found a nonsignificant 21% reduction in mortality from breast carcinoma (RR: 0.79, p = 0.14) by the Endpoint Committee (EPC) model, and a borderline significant 23% rate reduction was observed using the swedish cause of death register (SCB) follow-up model (RR: 0.77, p = 0.05).

Table 5 shows screening details of RCTs using MMG.

COCHRANE REVIEW[20,21]

This landmark review carried out by Olsen and Gøtzsche classified the trials into two groups: (1) Adequately randomized and (2) inadequately randomized **(Table 6)**.

When considering only adequately randomized trials, there was no reduction in breast cancer mortality at 7 or 13 years (RR: 0.90, CI: 0.79–1.02) when incorporating inadequately randomized trials, both 7- and 13-year reductions in breast cancer mortality significantly decreased (RR: 0.75). The overall RR for all seven trials was 0.81.

TABLE 6: Classification of trials.

Adequately randomized	*Suboptimally randomized*
Malmö I trial	New York HIP trial
Canadian trial	Malmö II trial
UK age trial	Swedish Two-County trial
	Göteborg trial
	Stockholm trial
	Edinburgh trial—not included

Their conclusion emphasized that breast cancer mortality is an unreliable outcome and biased in favor of screening and although the studies lacked the statistical power to assess all-cause mortality, no benefit in all-cause mortality was observed with screening MMG across all age groups, regardless of the kind of trial (adequately/inadequately randomized trial).

In conclusion, they highlighted that for every 2,000 women invited for screening throughout 10 years, one would avoid dying from breast cancer, while 10 healthy women, who would have remained undiagnosed without screening, would undergo unnecessary treatment.

Ultrasound

The combination of MMG and ultrasound for screening of breast cancer has shown an increased detection rate (improved sensitivity), which comes at a cost of unacceptable high false positives and increased biopsy rates. The addition of a single screening ultrasound to MMG in women with elevated risk of breast cancer will yield an additional 1.1–7.2 cancers per 1,000 high-risk women, but it will also substantially increase the number of false positives.[22] However, there is no study that shows a reduction in mortality due to the incremental value of ultrasound to MMG. It can at best serve as an additional tool to MMG screening in women with intermediate risk for breast cancer (personal history of breast cancer or biopsies associated with increased risk or relative with early onset breast cancer). The final assessment of ultrasound-detected lesions is also categorized using BI-RADS (Breast Imaging Reporting and Data System) scoring **(Table 7)**.

TABLE 7: American College of Radiology-Breast Imaging Reporting and Data System (ACR-BI RADS).

Categories	***5th edition***	***Likelihood of cancer***
Category 0	Incomplete—additional imaging needed	N/A
Category 1	Negative	Essentially 0%
Category 2	Benign	Essentially 0%
Category 3	Probably Benign	0 to ≤2%
Category 4	Suspicious	
4a:	Low suspicion of malignancy	>2 to ≤10%
4b:	Moderate suspicion of malignancy	>10 to ≤50%
4c:	High suspicion of malignancy	>50 to <95%
Category 5	Highly suggestive of malignancy	≥95%
Category 6	Known biopsy-proven malignancy	N/A

Magnetic Resonance Imaging

Magnetic resonance imaging has proven to be more sensitive than MMG for patients at higher-than-average risk for breast cancer. It is universally recommended for women who are breast cancer type 1 (BRCA1) or BRCA2 positive and for those with a higher than 25% lifetime risk of breast cancer. A German study[23] assessed MRI for supplemental screening in women at average risk of breast cancer (lifetime risk <15%) and found that MRI helped identify additional breast cancers that were not detected with MMG or USG, with a additional cancer yield of 15.5/1,000 cases. These additional cancers diagnosed were small (median size 8 mm), mostly node-negative (93%), and tended to exhibit an adverse biological profile. The interval cancer rate was 0%. They suggested the use of MRI as a supplemental tool in average-risk women, especially those with dense breasts.

Integration of Artificial Intelligence

The incorporation of artificial intelligence (AI) into screening MMG shows great potential in improving breast cancer detection, minimizing false positives, and streamlining the efficiency of breast cancer screening programs. A randomized trial conducted in Sweden[24] aimed to evaluate the clinical safety of AI-supported MMG screening compared to traditional radiologist interpretation. The study involved 80,033 women, and the AI-supported screening detected 244 cases of cancer at a rate of 6.1/1,000 participants, meeting safety benchmarks. In contrast, standard screening identified 203 cancers at a rate of 5.1/1,000. Notably, recall rates, false positive rates, and positive predictive values remained similar between the two methods. Furthermore, AI significantly reduced the workload associated with screening by 44.3%. This study demonstrates the safety and efficacy of AI integration in MMG screening, maintaining a comparable cancer detection rate while enhancing efficiency. The trial will continue to monitor interval cancer rates in a cohort of 100,000 participants during a 2-year follow-up period.

EFFECTIVENESS OF SCREENING

Downstaging

The aim of screening interventions is to detect the disease in the early stages and facilitate timely intervention and treatment. Most screening studies have demonstrated an increased incidence in the intervention arm compared to the control arm, with no difference in mortality. However, the lesions detected in the screened arm are typically early-stage breast cancers. The impact on breast cancer-related mortality can only be expected if the intervention can definitively demonstrate the downstaging of breast cancer.

Overdiagnosis

Over-diagnosed lesions refer to diseases that would never have become clinically apparent without screening before a patient's death. In an overview of seven autopsy studies, the median prevalence of occult invasive breast cancer was 1.3% (range, 0–1.8%), and of ductal carcinoma in situ was 8.9% (range, 0–14.7%).[25,26] Treating these cancers would be considered overtreatment.

Overdiagnosis is a significant drawback associated with MMG and CBE may offer respite to the same. Kalager et al.[6] pointed out that the amount of overdiagnosis observed in the previous randomized controlled trials is strikingly similar (22–24%). The concern with overdiagnosis is clinicians cannot identify which impalpable lesions detected by screening MMG will never progress within the lifetime of the women and thus must treat all diagnosed lesions. It may be argued that much of the overdiagnosis that occurs with MMG may be avoided by CBE alone. As the sensitivity of CBE is low, there is a possibility of false negative findings; however, given its high specificity, CBE tends to have low false positive rates.

Adverse Effects

While the efficacy and effectiveness of breast cancer screening have been proven by randomized studies, little attention is paid to the side effects of screening which are mainly due to false positive screen findings, necessitating further diagnostic imaging and biopsy rates. The psychological anxiety of a false positive finding and the morbidity of additional testing is also often ignored.

Cost Effectiveness

Determining the cost-effectiveness of CBE alone is difficult because no completed trial has really compared CBE versus no screening. Sarvazyan et al. reviewed the diagnostic accuracy, cost, and cost-effectiveness of breast cancer screening strategies worldwide. They concluded that in view of many countries with limited resources, more affordable strategies like CBE have the potential to provide effective screening for breast cancer.[27]

Table 8 highlights the various recommendations for screening.

CURRENT RECOMMENDATIONS

Overview:

- Awareness and self-breast examination as a tool for awareness in woman of all ages.
- No role of screening mammogram in women <40 years
- Annual clinical breast examination and awareness about breast cancer or Biennial MMG in healthy women over the age of 40 years.

TABLE 8: Recommendations for screening.

	ACR	*ACS*	*ACOG*	*NCCN*	*USPSTF*	*ACP*
Age to start MMG	40	45 with the option to start at 40	Offer at age 40 years, but no later than age 50 years	40	40	50, with a shared decision at age 40 years
Age to stop MMG	no age limit; should be tailored to individual health status	When life expectancy is <10 years	At age 75 years, screening decisions should be based on shared decision-making	Not stated	74	74 or in women with a life expectancy <10 years
MMG interval	Annual	Annual screening for individuals aged 45–54 years; annual or biennial for those aged 55 years and older	Annual or biennial	Annual	Biennial	Biennial

(ACOG: American College of Obstetricians and Gynecologists; ACP: American College of Physicians; ACR: American College of Radiology; ACS: American Cancer Society; MMG: mammography; NCCN: National Comprehensive Cancer Network; USPSTF: United States Preventive Services Task Force)

- However, the 25% probability of overdiagnosis must be kept in mind when recommending MMG as a screening tool. The additional biopsy needs for a facility for localization for impalpable lesions, related anxiety and referral to cancer centers need to be considered when advising a screening mammogram.
- High-risk individuals (BRCA positive, significant family history) to be treated as per standard guidelines.

CONCLUSION

- *BSE:* No evidence of reduction in mortality. Useful as an awareness tool.
- *CBE:* No published data on reduction motility. Effective in downstaging.
- *Imaging:* Reduction in mortality in women over the age of 50 years. Associated with 25% overdiagnosis. No mortality reduction in women <50 years of age.

REFERENCES

1. Bray F, Freely J, Soerjomataram I, Siegel RL, Torre LA, Jemal A. Global Cancer Statistics 2018: GLOBOCAN estimates of incidence and mortality worldwide for 36 cancers in 185 countries. CA Cancer J Clin. 2018;68(6):394-424.
2. Nagrani RT, Budukh A, Koyande S, Panse NS, Mhatre SS, Badwe R. Rural urban differences in breast cancer in India. Indian J Cancer. 2014;51(3):277-81.
3. Thomas DB, Gao DL, Ray RM, Wang WW, Allison CJ, Chen FL, et al. Randomized trial of breast self-examination in Shanghai: final results. J Nat Cancer Inst. 2002;94(19):1445-57.
4. Semiglazov VF, Manikhas AG, Moiseenko VM, Protsenko SA, Kharikova RS, Seleznev IK, et al. Results of a prospective randomized investigation [Russia (St Petersburg)/WHO] to evaluate the significance of self-examination for the early detection of breast cancer. Vopr Onkol. 2003;49(4):434-41.
5. Hackshaw A, Paul E. Breast self-examination and death from breast cancer: a meta-analysis. Br J Cancer. 2003;88(7):1047-953.
6. Kalager M, Adami HO, Bretthauer M, Tamimi RM. Overdiagnosis of invasive breast cancer due to mammography screening: results from the Norwegian screening program. Ann Intern Med. 2012;156(7):491-9.
7. Pisani P, Parkin DM, Ngelangel C, Esteban D, Gibson L, Munson M, et al. Outcome of screening by clinical examination of the breast in a trial in the Philippines. Int J Cancer. 2006;118(1):149-54.
8. Sankarnarayanan R, Ramdas K, Thara S, Muwonge R, Prabhakar J, Augustine P, et al. Clinical breast examination: preliminary results from a cluster randomized controlled trial in India. J Natl Cancer Inst. 2011;103(19):1476-80.
9. Mittra I, Mishra GA, Dikshit RP, Gupta S, Kulkarni VY, Shaikh HKA, et al. Effect of screening by clinical breast examination on breast cancer incidence and mortality after 20 years: prospective, cluster randomised controlled trial in Mumbai (published correction appears in BMJ). 2021;372:n256.
10. Shapiro S, Strax P, Venet L. Periodic breast cancer screening in reducing mortality from breast cancer. JAMA. 1971;215(11):1777-85.
11. Alexander FE. The Edinburgh randomized trial of breast cancer screening. J Natl Cancer Inst Monogr. 1997;22:31-5.
12. Miller AB, Baines CJ, To T, Wall C. Canadian National breast Screening Study: 2. Breast cancer detection and death rates among women aged 50 to 59 years. CMAJ. 1992;147(10):1477-88.
13. Miller AB, Wall C, Baines CJ, Sun P, To T, Narod SA. Twenty-five year follow-up for breast cancer incidence and mortality of the Canadian National Breast Screening Study: randomised screening trial. BMJ. 2014;348:g366.
14. Moss SM, Wale C, Smith R, Evans A, Cuckle H, Duffy SW. Effect of mammographic screening from age 40 years on breast cancer mortality in the UK Age Trial at 17 years' follow-up: a randomised controlled trial. Lancet Oncol. 2015; 16(9):1123-32.
15. Andersson I, Aspegren K, Janzon L, Landberg T, Lindholm K, Linell F, et al. Mammographic screening and mortality from breast cancer: the Malmö mammographic screening trial. BMJ. 1988;297(6654):943-8.
16. Zackrisson S, Andersson I, Janson L, Manjer J, Garne JP. Rate of over-diagnosis of breast cancer 15 years after end of Malmö mammographic screening trial: follow-up study. BMJ. 2006;332(7543):689-92.

17. Tabar L, Vitak B, Chen TH, Yen AM, Cohen A, Tot T, et al. Swedish two-county trial: Impact of mammographic screening on breast cancer mortality during 3 decades. Radiol. 260(3):658-63.
18. Frisell J, Lidbrink E, Hellström L, Rutqvist L-E. Followup after 11 years: update of mortality results in the Stockholm mammographic screening trial. Breast Cancer Res Treat. 1997;45(3):263-70.
19. Bjurstam N, Björneld L, Duffy SW, Smith TC, Cahlin E, Eriksson O, et al. The Gothenburg breast screening trial. Cancer. 1997;80(11):2091-9.
20. Olsen O, Gøtzsche PC. Cochrane review on screening for breast cancer with mammography. Lancet. 2001;358(9290):1340-42.
21. Gøtzsche PC, Jørgensen KL. Screening for breast cancer with mammography. Cochrane Database Syst Rev. 2013; 2013(6): CD001877.
22. Berg WA, Blume JD, Cormack J B, Mendelson EB, Lehrer D, Böhm-Vélez M, et al. Combined screening with ultrasound and mammography vs. mammography alone in women at elevated risk of breast cancer. JAMA. 2008;299(18):2151-63.
23. Kuhl CK, Strobel K, Bieling H, Leutner C, Schild HH, Schrading S. Supplemental breast MR imaging screening of women with average risk of breast cancer. Radiol. 2007;283(2):361-70.
24. Lång K, Josefsson V, Larsson AM, Larsson S, Högberg C, Sartor H, et al. Artificial intelligence-supported screen reading versus standard double reading in the Mammography Screening with Artificial Intelligence trial (MASAI): a clinical safety analysis of a randomised, controlled, non-inferiority, single-blinded, screening accuracy study. Lancet Oncol. 2023;24(8):936-44.
25. Welch HG, Black WC. Using autopsy series to estimate the disease "reservoir" for ductal carcinoma in situ of the breast: how much more breast cancer can we find? Ann Intern Med. 1997;127(11):1023-8.
26. Black WC, Welch HG. Advances in diagnostic imaging and overestimations of disease prevalence and the benefits of therapy. N Engl J Med. 1993;328(17): 1237-43.
27. Sarvazyan A, Egorov V, Son JS, Kaufman CS. Cost-effective Screening for Breast Cancer Worldwide: Current State and Future Directions. Breast Cancer (Auckl). 2008;1:91-9.

CHAPTER **10**

Optimizing IUI Results

Neelam Ohri, Namrata Ray Ohri

INTRODUCTION

In the era of rapidly advancing assisted reproductive technologies, intrauterine insemination (IUI) continues to hold a significant and valuable place in fertility treatment. Sperm preparation methods used for in vitro fertilization (IVF), such as washing, swim-up and swim-down techniques, and density gradients, have spurred interest in IUI.[1] Despite the popularity of IVF, IUI remains a less invasive and more affordable option for couples facing fertility issues. It is particularly beneficial for patients experiencing mild male-factor infertility, unexplained infertility, and certain female-factor infertility issues.[2] However, optimizing the success rates of IUI requires careful consideration of several factors, including appropriate patient selection, effective sperm preparation techniques, and meticulous timing and protocols for ovarian stimulation (OS).

FACTORS AFFECTING IUI SUCCESS RATE (FIG. 1)

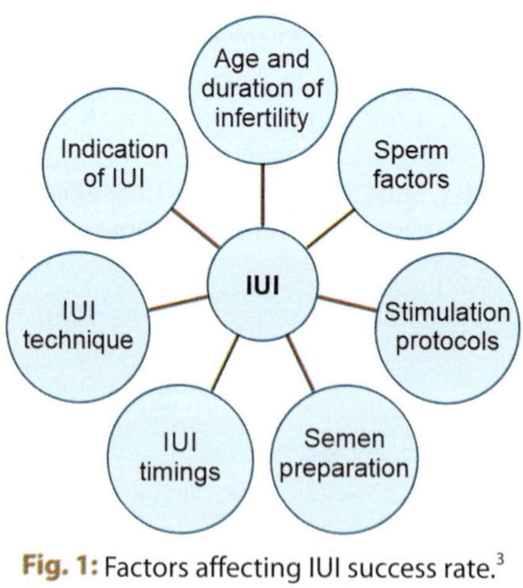

Fig. 1: Factors affecting IUI success rate.[3]

Patient Age and Duration of Infertility

As age increases IUI success rates decrease due to decreasing ovarian reserve. In women >35 years with antral follicle count (AFC) of <5, IUI is not indicated, and IVF should be considered.[4] IUI also has limited success when a couple has long-term infertility of >6 years.[5]

Cervical Factor

Massin et al. suggested performing IUI in spontaneous cycles in cervical indications when women are under 35 years old, and no male factors coexist.[6]

Endometriosis

In infertile women with revised American Society for Reproductive Medicine (rASRM) stage I/II endometriosis, clinicians may perform IUI with OS, instead of expectant management or IUI alone, as it increases pregnancy rates compared with expectant management. IUI with OS may be effective in increasing the live birth rate compared to IUI alone. Although the value of IUI in infertile women with rASRM stage III/IV endometriosis with tubal patency is uncertain, the use of IUI with OS could be considered. In these women, clinicians may consider performing IUI with OS within 6 months after surgical treatment, since pregnancy rates are similar to those achieved in unexplained infertility.[7]

Unexplained Infertility

It is often a tricky situation for the clinician as well as the couple when there is no obvious cause of infertility.

A Cochrane review by Pandian et al. has mentioned that IVF has a higher live birth compared to expectant management, unstimulated IUI, and IUI + gonadotropins, pretreated with clomiphene + IUI, but in treatment-naive patients, there is no conclusive evidence of a difference in live birth between IVF and IUI + gonadotropins/clomiphene.[8]

Semen Parameters

There are several parameters for semen to determine the success of IUI. In couples with unexplained infertility and men with a total motile sperm count (TMSC) of >10 million, at least three cycles of IUI with OS is the most effective option. Above a prewash TMSC of 3 million, IUI is less costly than IVF, and below a prewash TMSC of 3 million, intracytoplasmic sperm injection (ICSI) is less costly.[9]

Although, no distinct threshold of TMSC was identified to offer IUI versus proceeding with ART, there is a positive correlation between TMSC and IUI success. There appear to be improved outcomes with morphology >4% when TMSC <10.[10]

RECENT ADVANCES IN DIAGNOSTIC TOOLS FOR PATIENT SELECTION

Patient selection is an essential aspect of this treatment to yield better results.

Ovarian Reserve Testing

The AFC and anti-Müllerian hormone (AMH) testing provide a reliable assessment of ovarian reserve which is crucial for predicting response to stimulation and overall prognosis.

Tubal Patency Tests

Hysterosalpingography (HSG) and hysterosalpingo-contrast sonography (HyCoSy) are pivotal in assessing tubal patency. HyCoSy is less invasive and more comfortable for patients with good diagnostic accuracy.

Semen Analysis

Enhanced semen analysis techniques including deoxyribonucleic acid (DNA) fragmentation assays and computer-assisted sperm analysis (CASA), offer deeper insights into sperm quality apart from motility and count.

IUI CYCLE PROCESS

When a couple comes to the outpatient department (OPD), after thorough history-taking, examination, and investigations, pretreatment counseling must be done. This includes discussing the success rate, follow-ups, medications, cycle monitoring, and other important details and information of which the patient may be unaware.

The typical process of IUI cycle is given in **Flowchart 1**.

Flowchart 1: Algorithm for offering IUI cycles to couples.

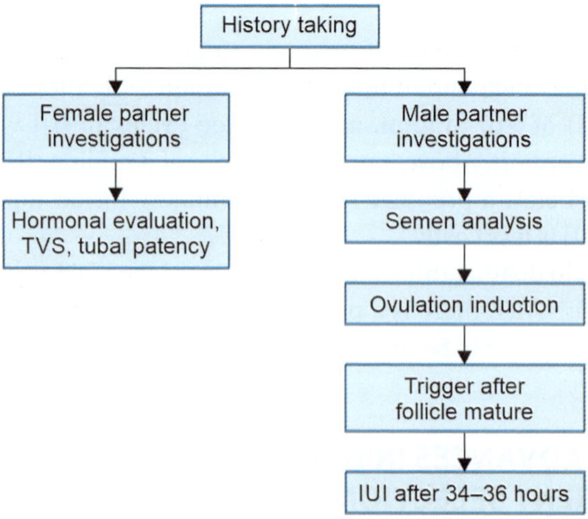

(IUI: intrauterine insemination; TVS: transvaginal sonography)

When the couple is received in the waiting area, paperwork and consent forms are completed. Then the male partner is sent for semen collection. After the semen sample is ready, sample verification is done, and IUI is performed. The patient rests for 15 minutes, and luteal phase support medications are prescribed.

OVARIAN STIMULATION PROTOCOLS FOR IMPROVED IUI OUTCOMES

Superovulation is for women who are subfertile and the aim in IUI is to recruit a maximum of two or three follicles.

Protocols used are:
- Natural cycle
- *Oral ovulogens:* Letrozole/clomiphene citrate/tamoxifen
- Letrozole/clomiphene citrate + gonadotropins
- Gonadotropins[11]

Clomiphene

It is used in doses of 50–100 mg from Day 2/3 of menses for ovulation.

Letrozole

It is a third-generation aromatase inhibitor with the advantage of mono-follicular development and lack of antiestrogenic effect on endometrium. According to the European Society of Human Reproduction and Embryology (ESHRE)/American Society for Reproductive Medicine (ASRM) guidelines, it is used as first-line treatment for ovulation induction in PCOS patients.

Recommended regimes are as follows:
- 2.5–5 mg/day from Day 2/3 of menses for 5 days
- Extended long protocol for 10 days in PCOS patients
- Single dose of 20 mg letrozole
- Step-up protocol[12]

Oral Ovulogens and Gonadotropins

A study by J Liu et al. in 2016 analyzed 8,893 cycles of IUI treatment. In ovulatory women, OS with letrozole combined with hMG achieved a significantly improved live birth rate. hMG stimulation resulted in a high risk for twins.[13]

Gonadotropins

In IUI, the most commonly used protocol is the fixed-dose protocol. A constant daily dose of 75–150 IU of gonadotropins is started from Day 2/3 of menses with USG monitoring. There are higher chances of multiple pregnancies in this compared to the use of oral ovulogens.

INDIVIDUALIZED PROTOCOLS

Tailoring stimulation protocols based on individual patient characteristics and previous cycle responses can optimize outcomes and reduce risks.

Monitoring and Timing Strategies

Cycle monitoring is an important aspect when ovulation induction is done. It is mainly used to assess the maturity of the follicle and endometrial preparation at the time of trigger. A baseline scan is to be done before starting ovulation induction for AFC, to rule out any ovarian cyst, endometrium, and other uterine factors. Serial transvaginal sonography (TVS) is done from Day 7/8/9 onward. Trigger given when follicle reaches 18–19 mm with endometrial thickness of >7 mm which is most conducive for pregnancy.

Gonadotropin-releasing Hormone Analogs

Gonadotropin-releasing hormone (GnRH) agonists as trigger: In 2014, Danish investigator Peter Humaidan suggested that GnRH agonist trigger as a substitute for traditional human chorionic gonadotropin (hCG) for the final oocyte maturation at the end of stimulation resulted in a significant reduction of ovarian hyperstimulation syndrome but robust luteal phase support was needed.[14] R Taheripanah et al. from Iran in 2017 performed a randomized controlled trial (RCT) on 110 infertile women in comparing 0.1 mg GnRH agonist (GnRHa) (Group I) versus 10,000 IU hCG (Group II) for trigger. They measured E2, follicle-stimulating hormone (FSH), and luteinizing hormone (LH) 12 and 36 hours after injection. An LH surge was detected in all patients. LH levels at 12 and 36 hours after triggering were higher in Group I and were washed out earlier than in Group II. The pregnancy rate was higher in Group I, but the difference was not statistically significant (26.9% vs. 20.8%, respectively $p = 0.46$). Also, the incidence of ovarian hyperstimulation syndrome was not different between the two groups ($p = 0.11$). There was a significant difference regarding the estradiol levels at 36 hours after triggering ($p = 0.00$). They concluded that the effects of GnRH on endogenous LH surge are sufficient for oocyte releasing and final follicular maturation. Pregnancy rates and ovarian hyperstimulation syndrome incidence were similar and suggested that GnRH agonists might be used as an alternative option instead of hCG in IUI cycles.[15]

Gonadotropin-releasing Hormone Antagonists

Antagonists are typically used in conventional OS protocols in IUI for postponing ovulation triggers for a day or two and avoiding work on weekends and also been used to allow a greater number of follicles to mature and enhance success rates.

In one of the largest trials, IUI was postponed using 0.25 mg GnRH antagonist, and no difference in clinical pregnancy rate (13.7 vs. 16.2%, $p = 0.371$) or in the ongoing pregnancy rates between groups (11.9 vs. 14.9%, $p = 0.271$) was found. They concluded that when IUI cannot be performed at the ideal date, it can be postponed for 2 days with the support of GnRHa treatment, with results that are not inferior to those of regular protocol.[16]

SEMEN ANALYSIS AND PREPARATION TECHNIQUES

Semen comprises of seminal plasma, spermatozoa, nonspecific debris, and microorganisms. Seminal plasma provides nutrition to sperm and helps in sperm penetration through cervical mucus, but it also contains prostaglandins which when inseminated can cause anaphylaxis.

Sperm preparation techniques:

- Direct swim up
- Pellet and swim-up method
- Density gradient
- ISO care—one step

Semen Collection

- The collection jar should be sterile and nontoxic.
- The name of the partner/husband should be written on the lid and the side of the container.
- Sample to be collected on the premises, ideally.
- Volume, viscosity, and presence of other cells should be noted.
- Allow the sperm sample to liquefy for 20 minutes. If it does not, pass it through a 23-G needle.
- A drop of semen is put on a Makler chamber and examined under a microscope. The number of sperm in 10 squares on the chamber grid is the count in million/mL.
- The number of motile sperms in the same squares is counted and the percentage of motility is noted.

Direct Swim Up

- Take a 10 mL round bottom plastic test tube and label it.
- Pipette 2 mL of culture medium.
- Gently pipette 1.5 mL of neat semen underneath the medium.
- Cap the test tube and put in an incubator for 30 minutes to 1 hour.
- Pipette the top layer and cloudy middle layer of supernatant and discard the rest.
- Supernatant used for IUI after checking the count and motility.

Pellet and Swim-up Method

- Take one drop and put it on Makler Chamber for counting and motility.
- Take 2 test tubes, label them, and put 1 mL sperm sample in each.
- Add 2 mL using media in each tube and mix.
- Centrifuge for 10 minutes at 1,500 rpm.
- Aspirate out the supernatant.
- Gently layer the pellet with 1 mL ushing media/culture media and place the tubes in the heating block or container, then place the block in a heater or incubator.
- After 30–40 minutes remove 0.5 mL of the supernatant from each tube to make it 1 mL and put it in another clean tube.
- Determine the count and motility of the supernatant in the Makler chamber.
- Supernatant is used for IUI.

It is simple and easy to perform and cost-effective, but it cannot separate morphologically normal sperms from abnormal ones. Moreover, centrifugation produces reactive oxygen species and can cause damage to the plasma membrane of sperms and some sperms might get trapped in the concentrated pellet sometimes.

Density Gradient

- Take one drop and put it on the Makler chamber to measure the sperm count and determine the motility.
- Take two test tubes and label them with patient ID.
- 1 mL of 90% sperm gradient is layered in each conical tube with a sterile pipette.
- 1 mL of 45% sperm gradient is then gently layered on top of it with another sterile pipette.
- 1–2 mL of sperm sample is then gently layered on top of the two layers. Care is taken not to add too many sample as it results in poor separation.
- Without disturbing the layers, the tubes are centrifuged at 300 g (1,500 rpm) for 20 minutes.
- The supernatant is then pipetted out and discarded leaving the pellet with as little of the 90% solution as possible.
- Take a new test tube and add 5–10 mL of medium to it and transfer the pellet to this tube.
- It is then centrifuged at 300 g for 10 minutes. The supernatant is pipetted out and discarded.

  Add 5 mL media and repeat this step.
- For samples with good motility, a swim-up procedure is now carried out in a 6 mL test tube, the pellet is layered with 1 mL culture medium and incubated for 30 minutes in a CO_2 incubator. The upper layer is carefully pipetted out in another clean test tube.

- For samples with poor motility, the pellet is gently layered with 0.8 mL culture medium and incubated for 60 minutes. The supernatant is carefully pipetted out in a clean test tube.
- Alternately, the pellet is resuspended in 0.5–1 mL of culture media or using media.
- It is then checked for motility and concentration and is ready for IUI.

Microfluidics

The microfluidic sperm selection (MFSS) device has emerged as a promising adjunct in assisted reproduction treatments (ARTs). It employs mechanisms of biomimicry based on the microanatomy of the female reproductive tract through strategies such as chemotaxis and rheotaxis which is often attributed to the theoretical reduction in sperm DNA damage compared to other techniques. A slight enhancement in ART outcomes was observed when using microfluidic devices for sperm selection, albeit without any statistical significance.[17] Various types of microfluidic devices are available and after sperm sorting the sorted sperm is analyzed by strict Kruger criteria and used for IUI. It is simple to use and does not require extensive training and sorted sample is available in 30 minutes, and this method removes the sperm damage associated with sperm washing and centrifugation giving an advantage over other methods.

Magnetic-assisted Cell Sorting Device

After the density gradient, magnetic-activated cell sorting (MACS) can be used to separate apoptotic sperm with high proportions of fragmented DNA from the rest, thus improving the overall quality of the seminal sample.

Apoptosis is a physiological process aiming to remove abnormal spermatozoa in order to maintain testicular homeostasis. Functional alterations of Sertoli cells or overactivity of testicular apoptotic processes (known as abortive apoptosis) can impair the elimination of apoptotic cells during spermatogenesis and consequently increase the number of apoptotic sperm cells in the ejaculate. In normal physiological conditions, apoptotic sperm cells with externalized phosphatidylserine residues on the plasma membrane can be recognized and efficiently eliminated in the female genital tract by phagocytes preventing the fertilization of the oocyte by a spermatozoon with alterations in its DNA integrity. This important sperm-selection process is inconveniently bypassed when ART sperm-selection techniques are performed, such as density-gradient centrifugation or sperm swim-up.[18]

IUI PROCEDURE SPECIFICATIONS

- Usage of properly sterilized equipment, avoiding chemicals in the procedure room.
- It is preferable that the IUI room is next to the laboratory or at least is in the same complex where the sample is being processed.
- The time interval between sample collection and insemination should preferably not be >1 hour.
- Instruments used are Cusco's speculum or Sim's speculum with anterior wall retractor.
- Minimum handling of the cervix is advisable but in case of difficulty, the anterior lip of the cervix can be held with Vulsellum. More handling might lead to a release of prostaglandins causing pain and uterine contractions.
- Vagina to be prepared with normal saline avoiding any antiseptic solution.
- The IUI cannula has to be loaded properly avoiding dead space with an insemination volume of 0.5–1 mL and attached to a 1 mL syringe. Various types of cannulas are available rigid and soft.
- Insemination is done slowly over a period of 1–2 minutes and then the cannula is slowly withdrawn to prevent gushing out of the insemination. Minimum insemination of 1 million motile sperm is essential.
- Patient is advised to be in position for 15 minutes.

LUTEAL PHASE SUPPORT

Luteal phase support has been studied extensively in the field of ART, IUI, and in recurrent pregnancy loss.

The luteal phase support is needed in IVF/ICSI cycles as there is disruption of the corpus luteum due to excessive levels of E2 by controlled OS and the use of GnRH analogs.[19]

In a study it was observed that the benefits of luteal support therapy with progesterone in terms of pregnancy rates were only in patients undergoing IUI when receiving gonadotropins for OI; women receiving CC did not seem to benefit from this treatment. But still, it is empirically prescribed for patients in all cycles.[20]

Rationale for progesterone:

- Endogenous progesterone deficits could have a negative impact on the evolution of pregnancy through inadequate endometrial preparation to implant, and inadequate immune response to fetal antigens.
- Morphological and physiological changes characteristic of the window of implantation, the time 5–10 days after the LH surge during which endometrium is most conducive to blastocyst implantation, if progesterone secretion is below physiological values, it does not take place.

- It is well documented that the maternal immune system recognizes fetal, paternal, and placental antigens, producing antibodies found in serum during normal ongoing pregnancy.
- Progesterone has an immunomodulatory effect, involved in the mechanism of immunological tolerance that allows the course of pregnancy.
- Progesterone also has uterine-relaxing properties and hence reduces uterine contractions.

The vaginal progesterone or dydrogesterone (20 mg/day) provides a more easy-to-use and convenient method than intramuscular (IM) progesterone for luteal phase support (LPS) in IUI cycles with comparable pregnancy rates. In a study, it was also demonstrated that 400 mg of vaginal progesterone suppository should be the maximum dose for LPS when compared with 800 mg.[21,22]

Most studies report that one IUI per cycle results in a pregnancy rate similar to two IUI procedures per cycle. In couples with a mild male factor problem, double IUI may increase the pregnancy rate.[23]

Resting supine after the IUI procedure may also be associated with higher pregnancy rates than those in patients who ambulated soon afterward.[24]

When to say no to IUI?

In a recent observational study of 29,021 patients with infertility, the efficacy and safety of three IUI cycles compared with 1 ART cycle as a first-line treatment of infertility was assessed. In women aged 18–40 years compared with three cycles of IUI, 1 cycle of ART was estimated to have a similar probability of live birth. In women aged >40 years, one ART cycle was associated with a higher probability of live birth than three IUI cycles.[25]

Women with high baseline FSH and E2 (>10–15 mIU/mL and >40 pg/mL, respectively) are unlikely to achieve a live birth after controlled ovarian hyperstimulation (COH)-IUI treatment.[26]

CONCLUSION

Optimizing IUI outcomes hinges on a multifaceted approach that includes precise patient selection, advanced sperm preparation methods, and tailored OS protocols. The success of IUI is influenced by factors such as patient age, duration of infertility, underlying conditions such as endometriosis, and semen parameters. Recent advancements in diagnostic tools, such as AFC and AMH testing for ovarian reserve, and innovative semen processing techniques like microfluidics and MACS, provide valuable insights and improve the efficiency of the IUI process. Additionally, the strategic use of luteal phase support with progesterone and the careful monitoring of the IUI cycle play crucial roles in maximizing the chances of conception.

By implementing these evidence-based practices and staying abreast of ongoing research, gynecologists can significantly enhance the efficacy of IUI treatments and offer hope to couples striving to overcome infertility.

REFERENCES

1. Yovich JL, Matson PL. The treatment of infertility by the high intrauterine insemination of husband's washed spermatozoa. Hum Reprod. 1988;3(8):939-43.
2. Cohlen BJ. Should we continue performing intrauterine inseminations in the year 2004? Gynecol Obstet Invest. 2005;59(1):3-13.
3. Barbieri RL. Female Infertility. In: Strauss JF, Barbieri RL (Eds). Yen and Jaffe's Reproductive Endocrinology, 8th edition. Philadelphia: Elsevier; 2019. pp. 556-81.e7.
4. Chang MY, Chiang CH, Chiu TH, Hsieh TT, Soong YK. The antral follicle count predicts the outcome of pregnancy in a controlled ovarian hyperstimulation/intrauterine insemination program. J Assist Reprod Genet. 1998;15(1):12-7.
5. Yavuz A, Demirci O, Sozen H, Uludoğan M. Predictive factors influencing pregnancy rates after intrauterine insemination. Iran J Reprod Med. 2013;11(3):227-34.
6. Massin N, Cedrin-Durnerin I, Hugues JN. Intrauterine insemination: spontaneous or medically-assisted ovulation? Gynecol Obstet Fertil. 2004;32(10):898-903.
7. Becker CM, Bokor A, Heikinheimo O, Horne A, Jansen F, Kiesel L, et al. ESHRE guideline: endometriosis. Hum Reprod Open. 2022;2022(2):hoac009.
8. Pandian Z, Gibreel A, Bhattacharya S. In vitro fertilisation for unexplained subfertility. Cochrane Database Syst Rev. 2012;4:CD003357.
9. Ombelet W, Dhont N, Thijssen A, Bosmans E, Kruger T. Semen quality and prediction of IUI success in male subfertility: a systematic review. Reprod Biomed Online. 2014;28(3):300-9.
10. Mathes MA, Kastrick EA, Gustin S. Postwash total motile sperm count effect on pregnancy outcomes in intrauterine insemination. Fertil Steril. 2020;114(3 Suppl):e384-5.
11. Cantineau AE, Cohlen BJ, Heineman MJ. Ovarian stimulation protocols (anti-oestrogens, gonadotrophins with and without GnRH agonists/antagonists) for intrauterine insemination (IUI) in women with subfertility. Cochrane Database Syst Rev. 2007;(2):CD005356.
12. Mitwally TF, Said SA, Galal W, Chan M, Cohen J, Casper RF, et al. Letrozole step-up protocol: a successful superovulation protocol. Fertil Steril. 2008;89(4):S23-4.
13. Liu J, Li TC, Wang J, Wang W, Hou Z, Liu J. The impact of ovarian stimulation on the outcome of intrauterine insemination treatment: an analysis of 8893 cycles. BJOG. 2016;123(Suppl 3):70-5.
14. Humaidan P, Alsbjerg B. GnRHa trigger for final oocyte maturation: is HCG trigger history? Reprod Biomed Online. 2014;29:274-80.
15. Taheripanah R, Zamaniyan M, Moridi A, Taheripanah A, Malih N. Comparing the effect of gonadotropin-releasing hormone agonist and human chorionic gonadotropin on final oocytes for ovulation triggering among infertile women undergoing intrauterine insemination: an RCT. Int J Reprod Biomed. 2017;15(6):351-6.

16. Gobernado J, Alvarez-Colomo C, Rodriguez-Tabernero L, Barrero L, Fernández-Gómez JMF, Schneider J. GnRH antagonist administration to postpone a weekend intrauterine insemination: a large cohort study from a public center. Reprod Biol Endocrinol. 2016;14(1):53.
17. Aderaldo FJ, da Silva Maranhão K, Ferreira Lanza DC. Does microfluidic sperm selection improve clinical pregnancy and miscarriage outcomes in assisted reproductive treatments? A systematic review and meta-analysis. PLoS One. 2023;18(11):e0292891.
18. Pacheco A, Blanco A, Bronet F, Cruz M, García-Fernández J, García-Velasco JA. Magnetic-Activated Cell Sorting (MACS): a useful sperm-selection technique in cases of high levels of sperm DNA fragmentation. J Clin Med. 2020;9(12):3976.
19. Fatemi HM, Popovic-Todorovic B, Papanikolaou E, Donoso P, Devroey P. An update of luteal phase support in stimulated IVF cycles. Hum Reprod Update. 2007;13(6):581-90.
20. Miralpeix E, Gonzalez-Comadran M, Sola I, Manau D, Carreras R, Checa MA. Efficacy of luteal phase support with vaginal progesterone in intrauterine insemination: a systematic review and meta-analysis. J Assist Reprod Genet. 2014;31(1):89-100.
21. Taş M, Uludag SZ, Aygen ME, Sahin Y. Comparison of oral dydrogesterone and vaginal micronized progesterone for luteal phase support in intrauterine insemination. Gynecol Endocrinol. 2020;36(1):77-80.
22. Azargoon A, Joorabloo G, Mirmohammadkhani M. Luteal phase support in intrauterine insemination cycles: a randomized clinical trial of vaginal versus intramuscular progesterone administration. J Reprod Infertil. 2022;23(1):33-38.
23. Ghanem ME, Bakre NI, Emam MA, Al Boghdady LA, Helal AS, Elmetwally AG, et al. The effects of timing of intrauterine insemination in relation to ovulation and the number of inseminations on cycle pregnancy rate in common infertility etiologies. Hum Reprod. 2011;26(3):576-83.
24. Saleh A, Tan SL, Biljan MM, Tulandi T. A randomized study of the effect of 10 minutes of bed rest after intrauterine insemination. Fertil Steril. 2000; 74(3):509-11.
25. Chiu YH, Yland JJ, Rinaudo P, Hsu J, McGrath S, Hernández-Díaz S, et al. Effectiveness and safety of intrauterine insemination vs. assisted reproductive technology: emulating a target trial using an observational database of administrative claims. Fertil Steril. 2022;117(5):981-91.
26. Kaser DJ, Goldman MB, Fung JL, Alper MM, Reindollar RH. When is treatment with clomiphene or gonadotropin IUI futile? Results of FASTT and FORT-T, two prospective randomized controlled trials. Fertil Steril. 2014;102(5):1331-7.e1.

CHAPTER 11 PGT-A

Hrishikesh D Pai, Rohan Palshetkar

INTRODUCTION

Preimplantation genetic testing (PGT) was first successfully done by Handyside[1] and since then has evolved leaps and bounds. It is a technique with the help of which we can identify genetic defects in embryos created using in vitro fertilization (IVF) prior to implantation and comprises two components—preimplantation genetic diagnosis (PGD) and preimplantation genetic screening (PGS) now recoined as preimplantation genetic testing for aneuploidy (PGT-A).

Pregenetic testing for diagnosis can be done for a monogenic (single-gene disorder) or for structural rearrangement.

- *Preimplantation genetic testing for monogenic (single-gene) disorders (PGT-M):* The aim of PGT-M is to achieve a pregnancy, which is unaffected by a particular genetic condition, such as any known heritable genetic mutation carried by one or both biological parents. It may also be used to select embryos, which have a specific genetic makeup like a compatible human leukocyte antigen complex.
- *Preimplantation genetic testing for structural rearrangements (PGT-SR):* The aim of PGT-SR is to achieve a pregnancy, which is not affected by a particular structural chromosomal abnormality such as translocation in a couple with a balanced translocation, or deletion/duplication.

Only unaffected or normal (euploid) embryos are transferred into the uterus, and it eliminates the need for postconception aneuploidy screening and diagnostic procedures (i.e., amniocentesis and chorionic villi biopsy), which may lead to a difficult decisions of terminating the pregnancy. Invasive antenatal diagnostic procedure even carries a small risk of abortion, which is eliminated with PGT conception.

WHO CAN BENEFIT FROM PREIMPLANTATION GENETIC TESTING?

- Women aged 35 and older because there is a concern about the genetic quality of their eggs[3]
- Women experiencing recurrent, unexplained pregnancy loss
- Women with more than one failed fertility treatment
- *Carriers of sex-linked disorders:* They can choose gender determination to prevent sex-linked disease.

- Carriers of single-gene disorders
- Couples with family history of inherited disease
- Those with chromosomal disorders

HOW IS PREIMPLANTATION GENETIC TESTING PERFORMED?

In order to perform PGT, embryos must be available for testing. The patient needs to go through a regular IVF cycle in which hormones (gonadotropins) are used to stimulate the ovaries to produce more than one egg. When the follicles reach a desired size, they are triggered with a human chorionic gonadotropin (hCG) injection, and the oocytes are then retrieved from these follicles under short general anesthesia. The procedure is done under transvaginal ultrasound guidance. Then the mature eggs (oocytes) are then injected with the partners or husbands' sperms and are allowed to grow in the laboratory up until the day on which a biopsy can be taken, i.e., Day 3 or Day 5.

During the biopsy, an embryologist can either do a Day 3/Day 5 biopsy. In Day 3 PGT, they take a single-cell biopsy and then send it for testing; in Day 5 PGT, they take a biopsy of trophectoderm (many cells) and then send it for testing. Once the biopsy is taken, the embryos are cryopreserved **(Figs. 1 to 3)**.

The genetic material from these cells is then amplified using whole-genome amplification (WGA)[2] and then tested using the newer techniques of array comparative genomic hybridization (aCGH) or more recently next-generation sequencing (NGS), which enables testing of all 24 chromosomes.

The report is then available after 7 days of sending the sample for testing if a Day 5 biopsy was sent and in 2 days if a Day 3 biopsy was sent allowing possibility of fresh transfer in a Day 3 biopsy. The risks and benefits of Day 3 and Day 5 embryo biopsy are listed in **Tables 2 and 3**.

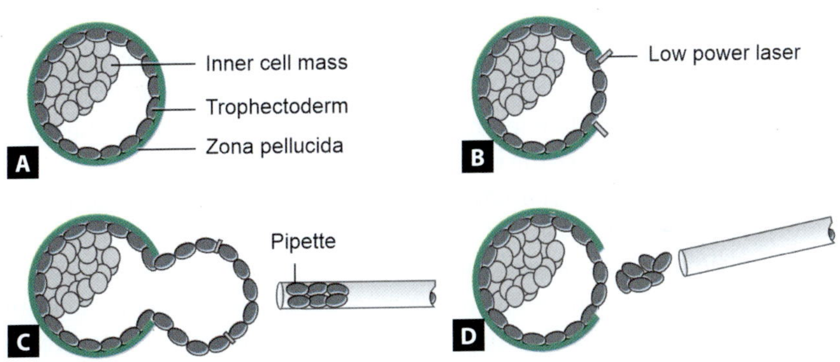

Figs. 1A to D: Steps involved in blastocyst biopsy. (A) Blastocyst; (B) Low power laser is aimed at the area on the trophectoderm avoiding the inner cell mass; (C) Taking biopsy from the hatched trophectoderm; (D) Biopsy completed.

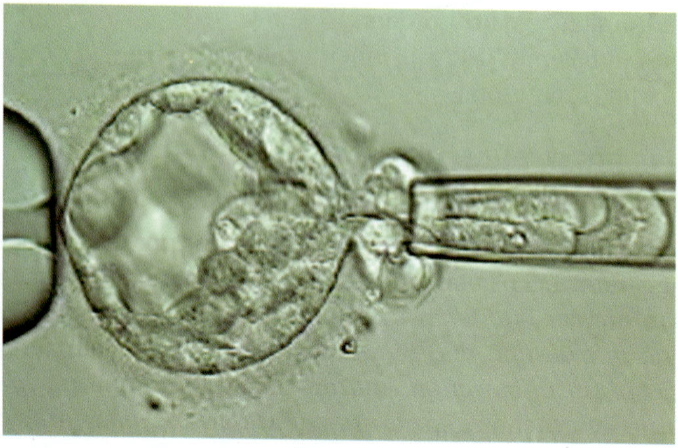

Fig. 2: Biopsy of the trophectoderm.

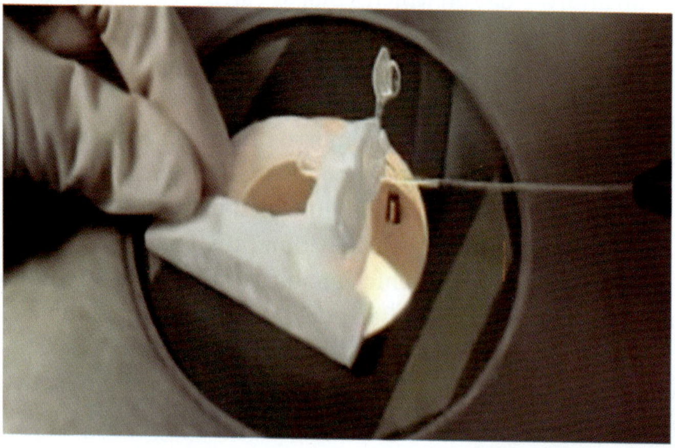

Fig. 3: Embryologist tubing a biopsy.

Depending on the report, a detailed counseling is mandatory for patients, especially if the report reflects Mosaic embryo. In a mosaic embryo, the chart shown in **Table 1** is used a reference while counseling the patient if the patient should or should not take the transfer of the embryo.

The report can show a normal (euploid), abnormal (aneuploid), or a mosaic embryo. In cases of mosaic embryo, a detailed genetic counseling should be done explaining the risk and the benefits of taking an embryo transfer **(Fig. 4)**.

Now-a-days, newer noninvasive pregenetic testing techniques such as analysis of cell-free DNA in embryo culture, and minimally invasive techniques such as blastocelic fluid aspiration are available.

But before you opt for pregenetic testing of any kind you should know the risks and the benefits.

TABLE 1: Reference for counseling a patient with a mosaic embryo on preimplantation genetic screening (PGS).

Mosaic chromosomes involved	***↑ Priority***	***Reasoning***
1, 3, 10, 12, and 19	Highest priority for transfer	Very low risk of any aforementioned adverse outcomes
4 and 5 and 47, XYY	The second group to be considered for transfer	Slightly increased likelihood of miscarriage or a viable aneuploidy (47, XYY)
2, 7, 11, 17, and 22	The third group to be considered for transfer	Slightly higher risk of miscarriage or a relatively low risk for uniparental disomy (UPD) trisomies 7 and 11
6, 9, and 15	The possibility for transfer should be considered with caution and only after detailed discussion with the prospective parents	Increased risk of miscarriage, UPD, or viable aneuploidy
2, 7, 11, 17, and 22	The third group to be considered for transfer	Slightly higher risk of miscarriage or a relatively low risk for UPD trisomies 7 and 11
8, 20, 47, XXX, and 47, XXY	The possibility for transfer could be considered after extensive discussion with prospective parents regarding the possible clinical manifestations	High risk of fetal involvement and a slightly increased risk for miscarriage and viable aneuploidy
13, 14, 16, 18, 21, and 45, X	Best avoided	Very high risk of any aforementioned adverse outcomes

TABLE 2: Benefits and disadvantages of Day 3 biopsy.

Benefits	***Disadvantages***
Provide information about both *maternal and paternal genotype*	*Fewer cells can be removed* for genetic analysis
Fresh embryo transfer after genetic diagnosis	• *High degree* of mosaicism • Chance of *impact on implantation rate* • Possibility of *not reaching the blastocyst stage*

BENEFITS OF PREIMPLANTATION GENETIC SCREENING

- Preimplantation genetic screening reduces the requirement for amniocentesis later in the pregnancy. Amniocentesis is prenatal testing done when the fetus is aged 10–16 weeks, where a needle is used to obtain

TABLE 3: Benefits and disadvantages of Day 5 biopsy.

Benefits	***Disadvantages***
Combining TE biopsy, blastocyst vitrification, and molecular analysis results in *high implantation and low miscarriage rates*	*Biopsied blastocysts need to be cryopreserved,* and they would be transferred in the next frozen cycle
Biopsy of multiple trophectoderm cells from the blastocyst *improves PGD outcome*	Effect on blastocyst developmental potential caused by TE biopsy would be *higher for blastocysts with less TE cells*
Reducing the risk of PCR failure and allele dropout (ADO)	*Experienced personnel* are required to perform the technique correctly and quantify the number of cells
Decrease of the incidence of mosaicism	

(PCR: polymerase chain reaction; PGD: preimplantation genetic diagnosis; TE: trophectoderm)

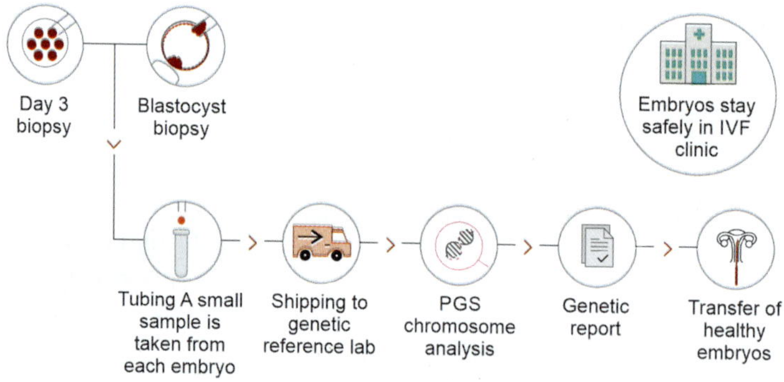

Fig. 4: Process from embryo biopsy to transfer. (IVF: in vitro fertilization; PGS: preimplantation genetic screening)

a sample of amniotic fluid. As it is invasive and carries some risk, having an option to avoid this test may be of valuable benefit to some patients.

- It enables the implantation of only selected quality preembryo(s). This increases the chances of getting pregnant and also decreases the chance of a miscarriage.
- It also decreases the chance of multiple births. Because they are screened for quality, fewer embryos can be transferred. It helps to identify the single best embryo and allows a single embryo to be transferred which in turn helps avoid the risks and complication of a multiple pregnancy and birth.

RISKS OF PREIMPLANTATION GENETIC SCREENING

Some genetic disorders may not show up until a later stage in life. PGD is highly effective, but in rare cases, a defective embryo may not show the disease or defect until mature.

CONCLUSION

Preimplantation genetic testing is a valuable adjunct to assisted reproductive technologies and plays a pivotal role in increasing success rates.[4] However, defining the exact benefit conferred by PGS and determining exactly which patient populations could be best served by PGS, however, are currently controversial. Despite the current lack of definitive data, PGS is increasingly being applied to patients with ever-expanding clinical indications. While there are few large randomized controlled studies defining the benefits of PGS, clinical data emerging from many PGS laboratories around the world is encouraging. Therefore, the judicious use of PGS seems reasonable at the present time, as the preponderance of available current evidence suggests that some couples may see a benefit from this technology.

REFERENCES

1. Handyside AH, Kontogianni EH, Hardy K, Winston RM. Pregnancies from biopsied human preimplantation embryos sexed by Y-specific DNA amplification. Nature. 1990;344(6268):768-70.
2. Harper JC, Wilton L, Traeger-Synodinos J, Goossens V, Moutou C, SenGupta SB, et al. The ESHRE PGD Consortium: 10 years of data collection. Hum Reprod Update. 2012;18(5):234-47.
3. Munné S, Chen S, Fischer J, Colls P, Zheng X, Stevens J, et al. Preimplantation genetic diagnosis reduces pregnancy loss in women aged 35 years and older with a history of recurrent miscarriages. Fertil Steril. 2005;83(3):722-7.
4. Scott RT Jr, Ferry K, Su J, Tao X, Scott K, Treff NR. Comprehensive chromosome screening is highly predictive of the reproductive potential of human embryos: a prospective, blinded, nonselection study. Fertil Steril. 2012;97(4):870-5.

CHAPTER 12 Internal Iliac Artery Ligation

Mahesh Gupta

INTRODUCTION

Internal iliac artery (IIA) ligation, also known as hypogastric artery ligation, is a surgical procedure used in various medical specialties, primarily in obstetrics and gynecology, to manage life-threatening hemorrhage originating from the pelvic region. This intervention involves the occlusion or ligation of the internal iliac artery to control excessive bleeding, particularly in cases of obstetric emergencies, pelvic trauma, or certain gynecological conditions. This write-up will explore the procedure, indications, and clinical implications of internal iliac artery ligation.

PROCEDURE

There are three approaches for internal iliac artery dissection, they are as follows:

1. Anterior approach
2. Posterior approach
3. Extraperitoneal approach

Internal iliac artery ligation is typically performed as an emergency procedure under anesthesia. The surgical approach may vary depending on the specific clinical scenario and surgeon's preference. However, it often involves a lower abdominal or pelvic incision to access the iliac vessels.

The author's approach is posterior in obstetric cases. Internal iliac artery ligation in obstetric cases means anterior division of internal iliac artery (IIL) always.

- The uterus is to be exteriorized after the delivery of the fetus and placenta.
- Abdominal content is packed with sterile mops.
- Infundibulopelvic ligament near ovary to be held by Babcock forceps, loose peritoneal fold lifted with artery forceps.
- Small cut with dissecting scissors and expand the incision with scissors up and down **(Fig. 1)**.
- Blunt dissection with fingers one can easily reach the bifurcation of the iliac vessel **(Fig. 2)**.
- The ureter is on a medial leaf of the peritoneum and can be taken with one more Babcock forceps to secure.
- 2–3 cm away from bifurcation (to avoid injury to the posterior division branch and injury to the iliac vein as it transverses more laterally as descends).

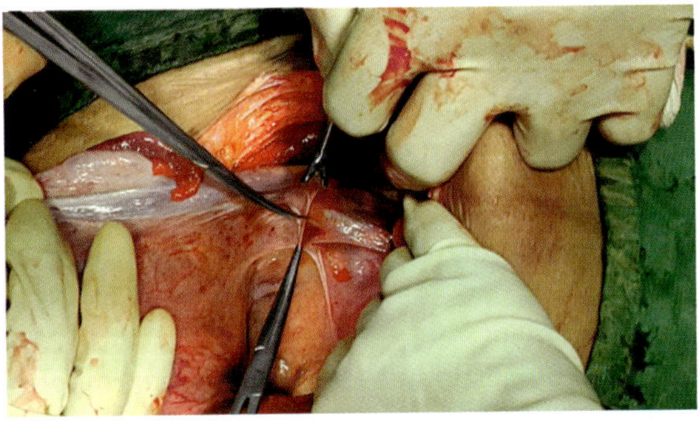

Fig. 1: Opening the peritoneum.

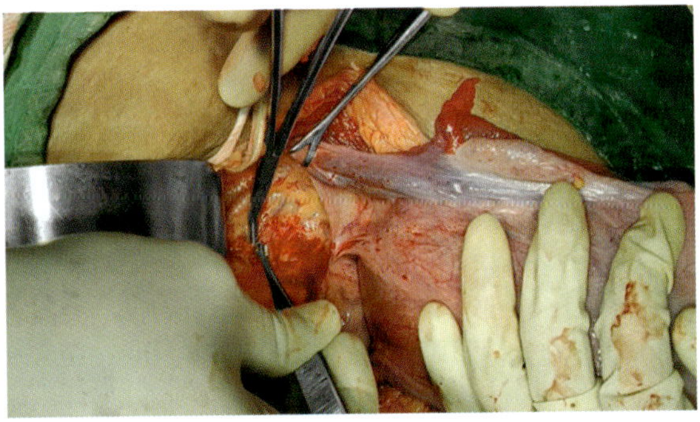

Fig. 2: Isolating the vessels.

- An important tip is to break the sheath of the internal iliac artery. This is the most important step for IIL.
- Once the sheath is broken pass the right angle forceps between the sheath and artery wall. Never blindly pass right angle forceps beneath the sheath means forceps should be between sheath and artery and not between sheath and internal iliac vein.
- Tie with delayed absorbable suture material like Vicryl No 1.
- For beginners, check for dorsalis pedis pulsation after IIL.
- Secure hemostasis and can keep peritoneal incision unsutured.

INDICATIONS

Internal iliac artery ligation is indicated in situations where conventional methods fail to control severe pelvic hemorrhage or when immediate and aggressive intervention is required to prevent life-threatening consequences. Common indications include:

Postpartum hemorrhage (PPH) has two parts:

1. Traumatic PPH

2. *Uterine organ PPH:*
   - Upper segment PPH (atonic PPH)
   - Lower segment PPH [placenta previa or placenta accreta spectrum (PAS) bleeding]

Traumatic PPH: This may be the only and sole treatment for traumatic PPH.

- Always a surgical means of treatment
- No dilemma
- No medical management
- Vaginal wall hematoma, supra levator hematoma, colporrhexis, rupture uterus, broad ligament hematoma, and uterine scar extension.
- Postobstetric hysterectomy hemoperitoneum

Atonic and lower segment PPH: May not be the sole and only treatment for organ PPH. But IIL can give additional security.

CLINICAL IMPLICATIONS

Internal iliac artery ligation is an effective technique for controlling severe pelvic hemorrhage, but it carries certain clinical implications:

- *Risk of ischemia:* Complete ligation of the internal iliac artery can result in ischemia to pelvic organs supplied by its branches, leading to potential complications such as buttock claudication, impotence, or bladder dysfunction.
- *Selective ligation:* Preservation of collateral circulation through selective or partial ligation techniques can minimize ischemic complications while achieving hemostasis. Careful patient selection and surgical planning are crucial to balance the risks and benefits of this approach.
- *Multidisciplinary approach:* Internal iliac artery ligation may require a multidisciplinary team involving obstetricians, gynecologists, trauma surgeons, and interventional radiologists to ensure optimal patient outcomes. Close collaboration and effective communication among team members are essential. But with enough experience, any gynecologist can perform it.
- *Postoperative monitoring:* Patients undergoing internal iliac artery ligation require vigilant postoperative monitoring for signs of ischemia, hemorrhage recurrence, or other complications. Close follow-up and appropriate management of sequelae are essential for long-term care.

CONCLUSION

Internal iliac artery ligation is a valuable surgical technique for managing severe pelvic hemorrhage in various clinical scenarios. While it carries certain risks and clinical implications, when performed judiciously and in appropriate cases, it can be life-saving and contribute to favorable patient outcomes. Close attention to patient selection, surgical technique, and postoperative care is essential to maximize the benefits of this intervention while minimizing potential complications.

CHAPTER 13 Acute Respiratory Conditions in Pregnancy

Priyankur Roy, Athulya Shajan

INTRODUCTION

Several anatomical and physiological changes to the respiratory system occur throughout a typical pregnancy. Several pulmonary illnesses may arise in the patient as a result of some of these changes. If lung diseases are not well managed, pregnancy may be compromised. This chapter discusses these anatomical and physiological changes as well as the clinical manifestation and management of lung illnesses that develop during pregnancy, both acute and chronic.[1,2]

CARDIORESPIRATORY PHYSIOLOGY AND PREGNANCY

Pregnancy-related changes to the respiratory system result in an increase in air volume and gas exchange, which improves the fetus's access to oxygen and its ability to exhale carbon dioxide. The expanding uterus, as well as hormonal and metabolic alterations, mediate these changes. Moderate respiratory alkalosis is the result of these modifications.[3]

Spirometry assessments of the forced vital capacity forced expiratory volume in 1 second (FEV1), and flow rates typically remain constant. Lung compliance remains unchanged throughout a healthy pregnancy. Toward the end of the first trimester, minute ventilation increases by 20–50% and stays steady the rest of the pregnancy.[4,5] The rise is associated with an increase in tidal volume rather than an increase in respiratory rate and is assumed to be brought on by elevated progesterone levels **(Fig. 1)**.

ASTHMA

Up to 8% of pregnant women experience asthma, making it one of the most prevalent respiratory diseases in pregnancy.[6] Chronic airway inflammation that is either fully or partially reversible is what defines asthma. Wheezing, dyspnea, coughing, and tightness in the chest are some of the signs and symptoms of asthma.[7] It is also linked to triggers, such as allergies, irritants, weather changes, stress, and exercise. Although the causes are unclear, asthmatic pregnant women are more likely to experience miscarriage, congenital defects, hypertension, preterm birth, intrauterine growth restriction, and low birth weight babies. Spirometry can be used to diagnose asthma in female patients who have no prior history of the illness.

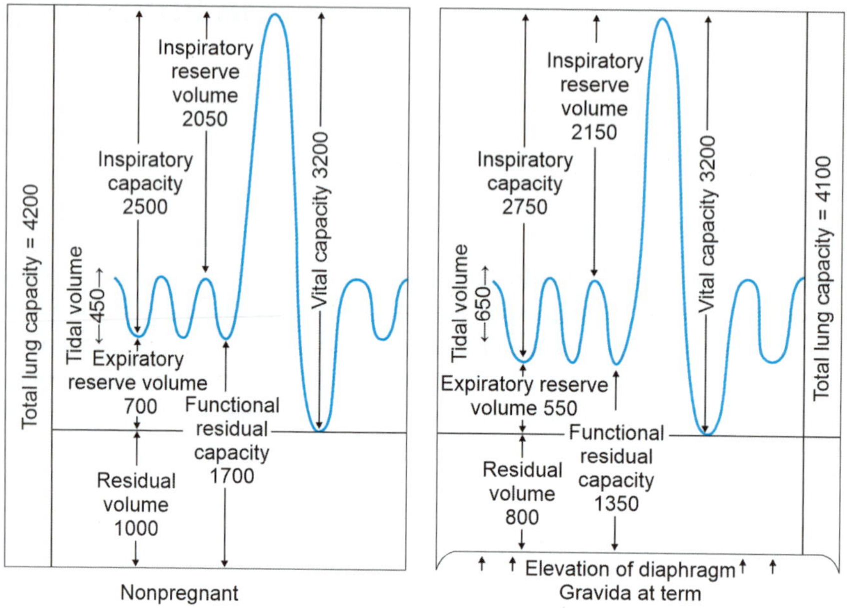

Fig. 1: The effect of pregnancy on pulmonary function. There is a gradual decrease in RV and FRC, while VC and TLC remain the same. (FRC: functional residual capacity; RV: residual volume; TLC: total lung capacity; VC: vital capacity)

Alternatively, if a woman's forced expiratory volume (FEV) improves by at least 12% after taking α-agonist, an asthma diagnosis is considered to have been made. Other differential diagnoses that could be made if asthma is ruled out include allergic rhinitis, gastric reflux disease, pneumonia, and bronchitis.[8,9]

The medication regimen should be reviewed, and pregnant women with asthma exacerbation should follow-up with a pulmonologist or a specialist in maternal-fetal medicine. To maintain ideal maternal oxygenation during the antepartum period, emphasis must be placed on medication compliance **(Table 1)**.[10]

For women who need maintenance at step 3 and above, clinicians may consult a pulmonologist or a specialist in maternal-fetal medicine.[11,12] Pregnant women diagnosed with asthma often cite "not wanting to harm the baby" as a reason to miss doses of medication, despite clinician reassurance. *The American Congress of Obstetricians and Gynaecologists recommends pregnant women diagnosed with asthma to continue with asthma medications rather than risk asthma symptoms or exacerbations.* Preventing maternal hypoxia and enhancing fetal well-being depend on ongoing patient education on following the recommended drug regimen throughout each antenatal appointment is the goal of therapy.[13]

TABLE 1: Progressive approach to medical management in bronchial asthma.

Drug category	SABA	LABA	ICSs OCS51	Systemic corticosteroids	Combinat on of ICS and LABA	Leukotriene agents	Anticholinergic	Anti-IgE
Examples	Albuterol nebulized solution, levalbuterol HFA, levalbuterol nebulized solution, and terbutaline	Formoterol and salmeterol	Budesonide nebulized/DPI, beclomethasone HFA, ciclesonide HFA, fluticasone I-IFA/Diskus®, and mometasone DPI	Medrol PO, and prednisone PO	Budesonide/ formoterol HFA, fluticasone/ salmeterol HFA/ mometasone/ formoterol FI	Montelukast tablets, zafirlukast, and zileuton tablets	Ipratropium HFA/nebulized solution	Omalizumab injectable

(DPI: dry powder inhaler; FI: fumarate inhalation; HFA: hydrofluoroalkane; ICS: inhaled corticosteroid; LABA: long-acting bronchodilator; OCS: oral corticosteroids; SABA: short-acting bronchodilators; long-acting bronchodilators)

PNEUMONIA

There are numerous microbes that might cause pneumonia in pregnant patients, but some of these microbes, such as viruses, fungi, and mycobacteria, may be more dangerous to pregnant women than others.[14,15]

Bacterial Pneumonia

In bacterial pneumonia, fever, chills, and a cough that produces purulent sputum are the most typical symptoms. The two most prevalent bacterial infections are *Haemophilus influenzae* and *Streptococcus pneumoniae* (pneumococcus). With an orally active antibiotic, ideally, one related to penicillin or a cephalosporin, the majority of community-acquired pneumonias can be managed in an outpatient setting. In the event that *Legionella* or *Mycoplasma* are a problem, erythromycin should be added. The fetal auditory system can be affected when gram-negative bacteria are treated with intravenous aminoglycosides. Tetracycline, which may disrupt fetal skeletal and dental development, and chloramphenicol, which may result in "gray syndrome" in newborns are among the antibiotics that should be avoided during pregnancy.[16-18]

Viral Pneumonia

Clinical symptoms due to influenza A infection include fever, coryza, headache, malaise, muscle aches, and cough, and typically go away in 3–5 days. Long-lasting chest symptoms should raise the possibility of worsening pneumonia. Although not all pregnant women should get the flu shot and it should be administered after the first trimester.

Pregnant women with varicella pneumonia have a higher rate of increased virulence, worse complications, and increased maternal mortality during the third trimester compared to nonpregnant people. The symptoms of pneumonia, which include coughing, dyspnea, pleuritic chest discomfort, and possibly hemoptysis, typically appear 2–5 days later. There may also be oral mucosal lesions. As a result of infection during the first trimester, varicella might result in congenital defects. Late-stage pregnancy infection can result in premature labor and perinatal infection, both of which have a high infant mortality rate. Acyclovir has been administered successfully to treat varicella.[18,19]

TUBERCULOSIS

Mycobacterial diseases have become more common recently, presumably as a result of rising human immunodeficiency virus (HIV) infection rates, an increase in immigration from endemic nations, and a deterioration in public health services. Spread is through inhalation. It is a typical granulomatous lesion and has lymphatic and hematogenous spread.[20]

Smoking, immunosuppression, silicosis, type 1 diabetes mellitus (T1DM), malignancy, and overcrowding are some of the risk factors.[21,22]

Clinical Features

Clinical features include influenza-like illness, chronic cough, hemoptysis, unresolved pneumonia, and weight loss. Signs are pleural effusion, consolidation, collapse, and hilar lymphadenopathy.

Diagnosis

Diagnosis can be made using:

- Microscopy of sputum—Ziehl-Neelsen stained bacilli
- Smear-negative tuberculosis (TB)—chest X-ray
- BACTEC™ culture
- LN biopsy for extrapulmonary TB or cartridge-based nucleic acid amplification test (CBNAAT)/GeneXpert

The Revised National TB Control Programme (RNTCP) has released a "National Strategic Plan (NSP) for TB 2017–2025" for the control and elimination of TB in India by 2025.

Treatment

- *First-line treatment of drug-sensitive TB:* 2-month (8 weeks) intensive phase (IP) with four drug fixed-dose combinations (FDCs) followed by a continuation phase of four months (16 weeks) with three drug FDCs.
- *For new TB cases:*
  - IP consists of 8 weeks of isoniazid (INH), rifampicin, pyrazinamide, and ethambutol (HRZE) in daily doses as per four weight band categories.
  - Continuation phase three drug FDCs, i.e., (1) rifampicin, isoniazid, and ethambutol are continued for 16 weeks. To prevent INH-related neuropathy add pyridoxine 10–25 mg/day.

ACUTE RESPIRATORY DISTRESS SYNDROME

Acute lung damage with acute respiratory distress syndrome (ARDS) is characterized by pulmonary edema and increased vascular permeability. A pulmonary capillary wedge pressure of <12 mm Hg, radiologic evidence of pulmonary edema, exclusion of cardiac reasons for pulmonary edema, severe hypoxemia requiring >50% inspired oxygen, and decreased lung compliance are the diagnostic criteria for ARDS. The overall fatality rate for ARDS in the general population ranges from 30 to 70%, with patients who have multisystem organ failure having the highest mortality rate.[23]

The goal of treatment is to get rid of the underlying cause while also providing supportive care, such as mechanical breathing, nutritional assistance, and hemodynamic support.[24]

CONCLUSION

Pregnancy symptoms such as physiological dyspnea and hyperventilation are frequent; although, they are typically innocuous and do not indicate a serious underlying pathology, there are several respiratory issues that can occur in pregnancy. During antenatal visits, a thorough history and physical examination can give the doctor a baseline of pulmonary function to ensure early diagnosis of cardiopulmonary abnormalities and execute prompt therapies where necessary. Ultimately, for women with pulmonary disease, effective screening, patient education, and appropriate therapies can enhance maternal-fetal outcomes.

REFERENCES

1. Whitty JE, Dombrowski MP. Respiratory diseases in pregnancy. In: Creasy R, Resnik R, Iams J, Lockwood CJ, Moore TR, Greene M (Eds). Creasy and Resnik's Maternal-Fetal Medicine: Principles and Practice, 7th edition. Philadelphia, PA: Elsevier Saunders; 2014. pp. 965-87.
2. Fishburne JI. Physiology and disease of the respiratory system in pregnancy: a review. J Reprod Med. 1979;22(4):177-89.
3. Ueland K. Maternal cardiovascular dynamics. VII. Intrapartum blood volume changes. Am J Obstet Gynecol. 1976;126(6):671-7.
4. Ratigan TR. Anatomic and physiologic changes of pregnancy: anesthetic considerations. J Am Assoc Nurse Anesth. 1983;51(1):38-42.
5. Contreras G, Guttierrez M, Beroiza T, Fantin A, Oddo H, Villarroel L, et al. Ventilatory drive and respiratory muscle function in pregnancy. Am Rev Respir Dis. 1991;144(4):837-41.
6. McGinty AP. The comparative effects of pregnancy and phrenic nerve interruption on the diaphragm and their relation to pulmonary tuberculosis. Am J Obstet Gynecol. 1938;35:237-48.
7. Bonica JJ. Maternal respiratory changes during pregnancy and parturition. In: Marx (Ed). Parturition and Perinatology. Philadelphia: FA Davis Company; 1973. pp. 2-19.
8. Baldwin GR, Moorthi DS, Whelton JA, MacDonnell KF. New lung functions and pregnancy. Am J Obstet Gynecol. 1977;127(3):235-9.
9. Gee JBL, Packer BS, Millen JE, Robin ED. Pulmonary mechanics during pregnancy. J Clin Invest. 1967;46(6):945-52.
10. Milne JA, Mills RJ, Coutts JR, Macnaughton MC, Moran F, Pack AI. The effect of human pregnancy on the pulmonary transfer factor for carbon monoxide as measured by the single-breath method. Clin Sci Mol Med. 1977;53(3):271.
11. Rees GB, Pipkin FB, Symonds EM, Patrick JM. A longitudinal study of respiratory changes in normal human pregnancy with cross-sectional data on subjects with pregnancy-induced hypertension. Am J Obstet Gynecol. 1990;162(3):826-30.

12. Skatrud JB, Bempsey JA, Kaisen DG. Ventilatory response to medroxyprogesterone acetate in normal subjects: time course and mechanism. J Appl Physiol. 1978;44(6):939-44.
13. Rance K, O'Laughlen MC. Managing asthma during pregnancy. J Am Assoc N Pract. 2013;25(10):513-21.
14. Dombrowski MP, Schatz M; ACOG Committee on Practice Bulletins-Obstetrics. ACOG practice bulletin: clinical management guidelines for obstetrician-gynecologists number 90, February 2008: asthma in pregnancy. Obstet Gynecol. 2008;111(2 Pt 1):457-64.
15. Hasegawa K, Cydulka RK, Sullivan AF, Langdorf MI, Nonas SA, Nowak RM, et al. Improved management of acute asthma among pregnant women presenting to the ED. Chest. 2015;147(2):406-14.
16. Dombrowski MP, Schatz M. Asthma in pregnancy. Clin Obstet Gynecol. 2010;53(2):301-10.
17. McKinney WP, Volkert P, Kaufman J. Fatal swine influenza pneumonia during late pregnancy. Arch Intern Med. 1990;150(1):213-5.
18. Rodrigues J, Niederman MS. Pneumonia complicating pregnancy. Clin Chest Med. 1992;13(4):679-91.
19. Prowse CM, Gaensler EA. Respiratory and acid-base changes during pregnancy. Anesthesiology. 1965;381-92.
20. Mostow SR, Cate TR, Ruben FL. Prevention of influenza and pneumonia. Am Rev Respir Dis. 1990;142(2):487-8.
21. American College of Obstetricians and Gynecologists. Human immunodeficiency virus infections: ACOG technical bulletin number 169-June 1992. Int J Gynecol Obstet. 1993;41(3):307-19.
22. Bynum LJ, Pierce AK. Pulmonary aspiration of gastric contents. Am Rev Respir Dis. 1976;114(6):1129-36.
23. Rinaldo JE. Adult respiratory distress syndrome. In: Rippe JM, Irwin RS, Alpert JS, et al. (Eds). Intensive Care Medicine. Boston: Little, Brown & Co; 1991. p. 476.
24. Erickson NL, Parisi VM. Adult respiratory distress syndrome and pregnancy. Semin Perinatol. 1990;14:68-78.

CHAPTER 14

Pelvic Cancer Screening in Modern India

Bhagyalaxmi Nayak, Annith Kumar VM

INTRODUCTION

The number of new cases of cancer, a significant global health concern, is expected to increase significantly, from 18.1 million in 2018 to an estimated 27 million by 2040. Population growth, aging demographics, and changing risk factors are major contributors to this worrying trend, particularly in nations with lower Human Development Index (HDI) scores. The World Health Organization (WHO) and the World Health Assembly (WHA) are among the international health organizations addressing this crisis by highlighting the need for increased efforts to promote health and cut the number of premature deaths from noncommunicable diseases (NCD), such as cancer, by one-third by 2030.

The burden of cancer is particularly high in India due to its large and diversified population. In 2020, the nation reported 1,324,413 new instances of cancer and 851,678 cancer-related deaths. With a total of 438,197 cases, breast, oral cavity, and cervix uteri cancers are the most common cancer types across all demographic groups. Even though there are affordable screening options for many malignancies, the shockingly low participation rates persist. This article looks at the situation of pelvic cancer screening in India right now, discusses the difficulties encountered, and suggests ways to improve these programs' efficacy.[1]

INDIA'S PRESENT SITUATION REGARDING PELVIC CANCER SCREENING

In 2020, 18.3% of newly reported cancer cases and 9.4% of all malignancies in India were attributed to cervical cancer, making it a serious health concern. Cervical cancer is still the leading cause of cancer-related deaths among women, even though its age-standardized incidence rate has significantly decreased from 1990 to 2016. This is especially true in rural areas where access to health care is limited, and late-stage diagnosis is common due to a lack of awareness.[2]

The World Bank-funded NCD intervention program of Tamil Nadu's Health Systems Project (TNHSP) has resulted in marginally increased screening rates among women aged 30 years and older. Additionally, Puducherry found that screening rates for cervical cancer were greater in rural than in urban areas.

In contrast, states with a high incidence of cancer, such as Arunachal Pradesh and Andhra Pradesh, exhibit minimal screening rates. For instance, in Arunachal Pradesh, where the age-standardized rate (ASR) is 27.7 per 100,000, the screening rate for cervical cancer was only 0.8%. Even with an ASR of 48 per 100,000, Andhra Pradesh had a very low rate of breast cancer screening. In Meghalaya, oral cancer screening was barely 1.2%, even though men's ASR was 78.5 per 100,000.

According to the National Family Health Survey 5 (NFHS-5), there is insufficient application of the National Programme for Prevention and Control of Cancer, Diabetes, Cardiovascular Diseases and Stroke (NPCDCS) guidelines. It is imperative to address stigma, socioeconomic inequality, and integration concerns. Raising public knowledge, providing healthcare training, and using social media to distribute education could all greatly increase the percentage of people who get screenings **(Table 1)**.[3]

TABLE 1: NFHS-5 data regarding cancer.[3]

	Urban (%)	***Rural (%)***	***Total (%)***
Ever undergone a screening test for cervical cancer:			
India	2.2	1.7	1.9
Among states or UTs:			
Median	1.1	0.6	0.8
Minimum-maximum	0.1–10	0–12.6	0.2–9.8
Ever undergone a breast examination for breast cancer:			
India	1.2	0.7	0.9
Among states or UTs:			
Median	0.4	0.3	0.3
Minimum-maximum	0.0–5.9	0.0–5.3	0.0–5.6
Ever undergone an oral cavity examination for oral cancer (women):			
India	1.2	0.8	0.9
Among states or UTs:			
Median	0.6	0.2	0.5
Minimum-maximum	0.0–10	0.1–0.6	0.2–10.1
Ever undergone an oral cavity examination for oral cancer (men):			
India	1	1.3	1.2
Among states or UTs:			
Median	0.6	0.8	0.9
Minimum-maximum	0.0–7.3	0.0–5.9	0.0–6.3

(NFHS-5: National Family Health Survey 5; UTs: union territories)

Human papillomavirus (HPV) infection is the main risk factor for cervical cancer. Early marriage, having several children, using oral contraceptives, maintaining poor genital cleanliness, and smoking are other risk factors. The Papanicolaou test (Pap smear), HPV deoxyribonucleic acid (DNA) testing, and visual inspection with acetic acid (VIA) are effective screening techniques for early detection. Every five years, the Indian Department of Health Research determines that VIA is the most economical screening technique available. However, there are a lot of challenges in using and putting these screening techniques into practice.

OBSTACLES IN THE SCREENING OF PELVIC CANCER[4]

Low Rates of Participation

The poor participation rate in pelvic cancer screening in India is one of the biggest obstacles. Only 1.9% of women have had a cervical cancer screening, 0.9% have had a breast examination, and 0.9% have taken part in an oral cancer screening, according to the NFHS-5. These numbers draw attention to a significant weakness in the screening programs that are currently in place and emphasize the need for better outreach and engagement techniques. A number of issues, such as a lack of knowledge, anxiety about receiving a cancer diagnosis, and cultural stigma associated with the disease, frequently contribute to low participation rates.

Gaps in Socioeconomic Status

The use of cancer screening services is highly impacted by socioeconomic differences. Due to low literacy rates, difficult access to healthcare facilities, and the high expense of screening and treatment, women living in rural and economically disadvantaged areas are less likely to take part in screening programs. Poor families are frequently disproportionately affected financially by cancer diagnosis and treatment, which makes it difficult for them to pay for essential medical care.

Social Stigma and Lack of Knowledge

The lack of knowledge regarding the advantages of screening and the significance of early detection is a significant obstacle to cancer screening. Reluctance to undergo screening is also influenced by cultural beliefs and social shame in many societies. Since cancer is frequently regarded as a taboo topic, open discussion about it may be awkward or even prohibited in some cultural circumstances. A lack of knowledge and this stigma keep many women from looking for screening programs or enrolling in them.

Insufficient Infrastructure for Health Care

Many regions of India lack the infrastructure for a universal cancer screening program. There is a scarcity of qualified medical personnel, and many health centers are devoid of the tools and resources needed to carry out screenings efficiently. This problem is made worse by the differences in healthcare services between urban and rural areas, where resources and facilities are frequently insufficient.[5]

CRUCIAL COMPONENTS OF EFFECTIVE SCREENING PROGRAMS

In order to successfully address these obstacles and execute population-based cancer screening initiatives, several crucial elements must be established:[6]

Explicit Policy Formulation

For screening programs to be implemented and sustained, a clear policy framework is essential. This entails defining the target demographic, age ranges, recruitment tactics, screening techniques, and follow-up protocols. Policies ought to cover performance indicators, insurance plans, and funding as well.

Screening as a Methodology

A comprehensive care plan that involves prompt referral, diagnostic testing, and treatment also includes effective screening. Coordination is needed at the facility, community, and individual levels. Achieving successful results requires ensuring patient adherence and removing obstacles to screening.

Robust Infrastructure

It is imperative to have a sturdy health system with trained staff, organizational resources, and well-coordinated service delivery. To track and assess the program's advancement, this entails having qualified healthcare professionals, sufficient equipment, and effective data management methods.

Systems for Monitoring and Assessment

To ensure that screening programs continue to be both high-quality and efficacious, regular monitoring and assessment are essential. Setting quality standards, addressing contextual factors that could have an impact on the program's success, and gathering and evaluating data on key performance indicators are all part of this process.

Community Involvement

Educating the public about cancer and the advantages of early detection through targeted programs and education can boost participation rates.

Participating communities in the development and execution of screening initiatives contribute to the provision of accessible and culturally acceptable services.

Implementation Science Research

Policy and practice can be informed by studies that examine the viability and adaptation of screening programs in particular circumstances. Demonstration projects and pilot programs can offer insightful information about practical approaches for expanding screening programs.[6]

METHODS FOR ENHANCING THE SCREENING OF PELVIC CANCER

Raising Knowledge and Inquiry

Improving participation rates requires educating the public and raising awareness of the value of cancer screening. Campaigns for public health should emphasize informing people about the advantages of early detection and the accessibility of screening programs. Reaching a large audience and promoting a preventive healthcare culture can be facilitated by utilizing social media platforms and conventional media. Workshops and education initiatives rooted in the community can also make a big difference in raising cancer awareness and lowering its stigma.

Fortifying the Infrastructure of Health Care

Cancer screening programs cannot be implemented successfully until the healthcare system is improved. This entails providing health centers with the infrastructure they require and making sure there is a sufficient supply of screening supplies. Investing in medical staff training to do screens and offer follow-up treatment should be part of the infrastructural investment in health care. Strong referral networks and prompt treatment following screening are two other essential elements of a successful screening program.

Establishing Structured Screening Initiatives

Since organized screening programs consistently target populations that are considered to be at-risk, they are more effective than opportunistic screening. Regular follow-ups and tracking of screening results are necessary for these programs to guarantee that those who have positive results receive prompt and appropriate therapy. To maintain high standards and meet screening criteria, centralized administration, oversight committee evaluations regularly, and cooperation among healthcare professionals are necessary when implementing organized screening.

Dealing with Social and Economic Inequalities

The goal of efforts to reduce socioeconomic gaps in cancer screening should be to increase the accessibility and affordability of screening services. Free or inexpensive screenings can be offered in underserved communities with the support of government-funded initiatives and collaborations with nongovernmental organizations (NGOs). Furthermore, expanding the reach and lowering obstacles to access for more women can be achieved by incorporating cancer screening services into currently running public health efforts, such as maternity and child health programs.

Vaccination Against Human Papillomavirus

A tried-and-true strategy for lowering the risk of cervical cancer is HPV vaccination. The WHO advises immunizing girls between the ages of 9 and 13 as part of a comprehensive strategy to prevent cervical cancer. The HPV vaccine's inclusion in India's universal immunization program may considerably lower the country's incidence of cervical cancer. The main goals should be to boost vaccination rates, deal with vaccine hesitancy, and make sure the vaccine is accessible in both urban and rural regions.

METHODS FOR SCREENING FOR CERVICAL CANCER IN REMOTE AREAS

Rural Registries for Cancer

One important tactic for enhancing cervical cancer screening in rural regions has been the creation of rural cancer registries. Launched in 1987 in Barshi, Maharashtra, the first rural cancer registry in India has played a significant role in enhancing early detection rates and increasing awareness of the disease. These registries have made a substantial contribution to lowering the death rate from cervical cancer by enlisting investigators to visit villages regularly in order to detect cases and invite symptomatic women to screening camps. Cervical cancer screening has been more widely available in rural India thanks to the establishment of additional rural cancer registries in the districts of Ahmadabad, Ratnagiri, Sevagram, and Sindhudurg.

The Screening Camp

Using Pap smears as the primary method of cytological screening, screening camps are set-up in rural regions as part of the camp-based strategy. Studies have revealed that encouraging women to participate does not necessarily require just setting up camps. For instance, despite the availability of mobile cancer detection vans, the acceptance rate for Pap smear screening was only 8.3% in Barshi Tehsil, Maharashtra. Counseling and educational initiatives before the camps are crucial for increasing participation. Research conducted in New Delhi and Kerala has shown that regular interval screenings conducted through camps, when paired with the efforts of community volunteers, can increase the rates of involvement.

Village Health Nurses' Participation

It has been successful in rural areas in training village health nurses (VHNs) to recognize cervical lesions and conduct Pap smears. A 2-year initiative in Tamil Nadu that trained 101 VHNs led to the screening of 6,459 eligible women, and the program's success rate in obtaining sufficient Pap smears was 80%. Increasing coverage and guaranteeing routine follow-ups are important tasks for VHNs, especially in places where access to medical services is restricted.

Methods of Visual Inspection

A quick and inexpensive diagnostic substitute for cytology is visual inspection techniques, such as VIA and visual inspection with Lugol's iodine (VILI). These techniques are especially helpful in places with limited resources and cytological infrastructure. The benefits of VIA and VILI include same-visit treatment and fast results. Rural populations in Uttar Pradesh have discovered that VIA and VILI are practical primary screening techniques for identifying high-grade cervical intraepithelial neoplasia (CIN).

Using a Cytological Screen

Pap smears are still the gold standard for cytological screening, which finds preinvasive cervical cancer lesions. Cytological screening can reduce the incidence of cervical cancer by 80%, but its efficacy is limited in rural regions because of a lack of hygienic conditions and recurring vaginal infections. Studies from Lucknow and other rural regions show a high incidence of squamous intraepithelial lesions (SILs), which emphasizes the need for more comprehensive cytological screening and awareness campaigns. Frequent cytological screening is crucial, especially for low-income women who are more likely to acquire cervical cancer.

Human Papillomavirus-Deoxyribonucleic Acid Analysis

A highly specific and sensitive technique for cervical cancer early diagnosis is HPV-DNA detection. Research indicates that HPV testing, as opposed to Pap smears, can identify a greater percentage of CIN and cancer cases.

CONCLUSION

India's scenario for pelvic cancer screening is complicated, with many potential and obstacles. Notwithstanding the prevalence of efficient screening techniques and noteworthy progressions in cancer research, the nation has challenges related to poor involvement rates, socioeconomic inequality, insufficient awareness, and inadequate healthcare infrastructure.

To tackle these obstacles, a diverse strategy is needed. Raising public knowledge and educating the public is essential to raising participation rates and lessening the stigma attached to cancer. Enhancing the accessibility and efficacy of screening services can be achieved by fortifying the healthcare infrastructure with improved tools, skilled workers, and well-structured screening initiatives. By putting socioeconomic disparity strategies into practice, underprivileged groups will be guaranteed access to treatment without having to worry about paying for it.

Novel strategies like camp-based screening, rural cancer registries, and the use of VHNs have demonstrated promise in raising screening rates and promoting early diagnosis in rural settings. To solve cytological infrastructure constraints, visual inspection techniques and HPV-DNA testing offer useful options that can be included in current screening frameworks.

The inclusion of HPV vaccination in India's comprehensive immunization program presents a noteworthy prospect to mitigate the prevalence of cervical cancer and enhance current screening initiatives. A coordinated effort from governmental organizations, healthcare providers, and community organizations is necessary to fully realize the promise of these measures.

India may significantly lower the incidence and death of pelvic malignancies by tackling these issues and putting into practice comprehensive policies catered to the particular requirements of its diverse population. In the end, ensuring that screening programs are efficient, fair, and easily accessible will help to improve health outcomes and lower the national cancer burden.

REFERENCES

1. India State-Level Disease Burden Initiative Cancer Collaborators. The burden of cancers and their variations across the states of India: the Global Burden of Disease Study 1990–2016. Lancet Oncol. 2018;19(10):1289-306.
2. National Centre for Disease Informatics and Research. (2020). Report of National Cancer Registry Programme (ICMR-NCDIR). [Online] Available from https://www.ncdirindia.org/All_Reports/Report_2020/default.aspx [Last accessed August, 2024].
3. Thulaseedharan J, Gopika M, Prabhu P. Status of cancer screening in India: an alarm signal from the National Family Health Survey (NFHS-5). J Family Med Prim Care. 2022;11(11):7303-7.
4. Mehrotra R, Yadav K. Cervical Cancer: Formulation and Implementation of Govt of India Guidelines for Screening and Management. Indian J Gynecol Oncol. 2022;20(1):4.
5. Srivastava AN, Misra JS, Srivastava S, Das BC, Gupta S. Cervical cancer screening in rural India: status and current concepts. Indian J Med Res. 2018;148(6):687-96.
6. Sivaram S, Majumdar G, Perin D, Nessa A, Broeders M, Lynge E, et al. Population-based cancer screening programmes in low-income and middle-income countries: regional consultation of the International Cancer Screening Network in India. Lancet Oncol. 2018;19(2):e113-22.

CHAPTER 15

Fetal Growth Restriction: Delivery Decision Making

Abha Rani Sinha, Vinita Kumari

INTRODUCTION

Fetal growth restriction (FGR) also known as intrauterine growth restriction (IUGR) is a condition in which the fetus has not achieved its genetic growth potential due to some pathological factor irrespective of fetal size and is associated with a variety of adverse perinatal outcomes. The real challenge is differentiating constitutionally small fetuses from pathologically small ones.

There is a lack of consensus regarding terminology, etiology, diagnostic criteria, optimal management, and delivery timing for growth-restricted fetuses.[1]

Small for gestational age (SGA) is often used as a proxy for FGR. SGA is defined as an estimated fetal weight (EFW) or abdominal circumference (AC) less than the 10th centile and severe SGA is EFW or AC less than the 3rd centile. In contrast, FGR is defined as SGA with abnormal Doppler studies. Though the SGA fetuses are at an increased risk of perinatal mortality and morbidity, the majority of the adverse outcomes are encountered in the growth-restricted group.

Fetal growth restriction raises high concern as it is the leading cause of stillbirth, perinatal mortality, preterm births, and intrapartum asphyxia. It is also associated with neonatal complications, including meconium aspiration, cognitive dysfunction, cerebral palsy, and metabolic and hematological disorders.[2] In 2016, an international panel of experts on FGR undertook a Delphi procedure and agreed on a consensus, definition of early and late FGR with 32 weeks as the cut-off to differentiate between early and late FGR.

In the absence of definitive treatment of FGR, the management option is fetal surveillance and identification of delivery threshold.

Appropriate Surveillance, monitoring, and their expert interpretation in identifying fetal deterioration and eminent stillbirth is the cornerstone of the management of an FGR baby.

The main challenge in considering delivery in an IUGR fetus under surveillance is the risk of deterioration leading to stillbirth versus the risk of mortality and morbidity associated with preterm delivery. The tools used for monitoring will in discussed in the following section and their results raising alarm will be discussed in the following section.

MONITORING

The objective behind fetal monitoring is to prevent stillbirth. The monitoring tool should be efficient enough to diagnose fetal compromise and risk of imminent stillbirth necessitating immediate delivery.

Further going down the tools should be able to predict detection of fetal deterioration that precedes irreversible compromise. To achieve this goal, monitoring tests need to be accurate in identifying fetal risks that favor delivery.[3]

In cases where monitoring results permit deferring delivery, further monitoring frequency should be able to prevent adverse pregnancy outcomes.

Fetal surveillance includes maternal monitoring of fetal movements by the mother, cardiotocography (CTG), amniotic fluid volume, and fetal activity assessment by ultrasonography (USG) and Doppler ultrasound of the fetal arterial and venous circulations.[3]

FETAL MOVEMENT COUNTING

- Progressive fetal hypoxemia leads to decreased fetal movement.
- This can be perceived by the mother if she lies down and pays focused attention.[4]
- The "count to 10" method is followed where instructions for the woman to count fetal movements at the same time each day. If there are <10 movements in a 2–3-hour period after focused maternal counting it should be reported.[5]
- Fetal movement counting is an inexpensive tool to monitor fetal wellbeing in between regular checkups in the comforts of home and can be used as an adjunct to other monitoring methods.

FETAL BIOMETRY

Serial fetal biometry can detect fetuses with worsening FGR growth velocity measurements should be used 3 weeks apart to minimize false positives.[6]

DOPPLER ASSESSMENT

Umbilical Artery Doppler

Umbilical artery (UA) Doppler gives an indication of the hemodynamic status of placental function and hence is universally recommended for monitoring of FGR. It is used for outcome prediction of early-onset IUGR but does not reliably predict late-onset IUGR outcome. With increasing degrees of placental blood flow resistance, an abnormal UA waveform is defined as either having an elevated pulsatility index (PI), absent end-diastolic velocity (AEDV), or reversed end-diastolic velocity (REDV).[3]

The risk of stillbirth once AEDV develops is 6.8 and 19% once REDV develops but this risk falls drastically if intensive surveillance is done. It falls to 0–1% in the case of AEDV and 1–2% in the case of REDV.[7]

When the UA-PI increases but the end-diastolic forward flow is present, surveillance should be done twice a week but when AEDV develops, surveillance is recommended twice a week, and when REDV develops three times a week unless delivered.[3,8,9]

Cerebral Artery Doppler for Late Intrauterine Growth Restriction

Middle cerebral artery (MCA) Doppler gives an indication of placental dysfunction in late-onset FGR MCA is recommended for monitoring in late-onset FGR. Concurrent measurement of the UA and middle cerebral artery PI allows calculation of the cerebroplacental Doppler ratio (CPR). Both the cerebroplacental ratio and middle cerebral artery PI decrease in placental dysfunction, even with normal UA Doppler. In cases of decreased MCA PI twice-weekly surveillance is recommended due to adverse outcomes in 1 week.[10]

Ductus Venosus Doppler

In patients that do not yet meet delivery criteria, ductus venosus (DV) Doppler is recommended at a minimum of twice weekly in patients with AEDV and three times weekly when REDV is observed.[3]

Abnormal DV Doppler is primarily observed in early-onset FGR and can provide an estimate of fetal acid-base balance and the risk of stillbirth.[11]

The DV Doppler flow velocity pattern reflects atrial pressure-volume changes during the cardiac cycle. An increased PI and a retrograde a-wave in the DV reflect the onset of overt cardiac compromise, due to hypoxia and acidemia.[8]

AMNIOTIC FLUID VOLUME

Oligohydramnios can be defined as the sum of the four-quadrant amniotic fluid index below or equal to 5 cm, or a maximum single vertical amniotic fluid pocket below or equal to 2 cm. Use of the largest single vertical pocket is preferred as it reduces overdiagnosis of oligohydramnios.[12]

BIOPHYSICAL PROFILE

The five-component biophysical profile (BPP) comprises of CTG/nonstress test (NST) and maximum amniotic fluid pocket, fetal breathing movements, gross body movements, and tone, and therefore includes four indicators of short-term acid-base balance.[13] All five components of the BPP are assigned a score of 2 for its presence and 0 for its absence. Scores of 8–10 are considered normal 6 equivocal and 4 or less are abnormal. A BPP score <4 is an absolute indication of delivery. However, many studies suggest BPP as a poor predictor of fetal acid anemia in severely preterm FGR fetuses. Therefore, it is recommended that BPP not be used for fetal surveillance in preterm SGA fetuses.[14,15]

Cardiotocography

- Conventional CTG is not recommended due to inter- and intraobserver variation.[16]

- Computerized cardiotocography (cCTG) is recommended due to consistency.

A short-term variation ≤3 ms in cCTG has been associated with and grave prognosis and <2.6 ms is an absolute indication for delivery irrespective of gestational age.[3]

Surveillance Strategy

There is no consensus on a uniform surveillance strategy, but the aim is to prevent adverse fetal outcomes and stillbirth. The surveillance should be robust and a combination of available modalities so that accurate acid-base status is assessed avoiding unnecessary interventions and at the same time anticipate adversity, acidosis, and asphyxia.

Among these modalities, the combination of CTG/NST and UA Doppler is universally recommended.

When to deliver?

The most challenging decision in FGR is to decide when to deliver. In fact, each day in the womb decreases the risk of neonatal death, and major neonatal complications in a graded manner have to be, balanced against the risk of stillbirth in further continuing the pregnancy.

Gestational age is the most important criterion for neonatal survival. The decision regarding delivery requires caution, balance, and expertise in the interpretation of surveillance results.

ABSOLUTE INDICATIONS FOR DELIVERY

Absolute delivery criteria are monitoring and surveillance results that denote imminent grave risks to maternal or fetal health. Under such circumstances, a fetus is delivered irrespective of gestational age. Absolute indications for delivery at any gestational age and birth weight combination that are considered to be viable include: BPP or NST abnormalities.

Biophysical profile 60 minutes score ≤4- or 30-minutes score of 0–2 denotes severe fetal academia leading to fetal demise.

Repeated fetal decelerations, recurrent late bradycardia and loss of variability, and sinusoidal patterns or cCTG short-term variability (STV) <2.6 milliseconds are also associated with strong acid-base derangement leading to adverse perinatal outcomes and fetus should be delivered irrespective of gestational age.

In a suspected case of SGA or symphysis-fundal height (SFH) <10 percentile for gestational age after several measurements or EFW/AC <10 percentile for the gestational age monitoring should be done by:

- UA and MCA Doppler every once weekly/fortnightly
- Biometry/growth scan fortnightly

If these two are normal wait for >37 weeks and BPP/NST once or twice weekly is recommended. Such mild cases with no Doppler abnormalities can be delivered at term vaginally between 37 and 39 weeks.

In abnormalities, such as UA PI >95 percentile, PI or RI >2 SDs, MCA PI <5th percentile, CPR <5th percentile, oligohydramnios UA, MCA, and DV Doppler, and BPP/NST should be repeated once or twice per week and biometry fortnightly. If no further deterioration in surveillance results delivery should be considered at ≥34 weeks either by lower segment cesarean section (LSCS) or induction and vaginal delivery.

If the umbilical artery Doppler results show AEDV or REDV the situation is grave as the mean time of deterioration is 5 days in AEDV and 2 days in REDV. Hence monitoring has to be more frequent. BPP/NST has to be done twice daily and Doppler (UA, MCA, and DV) everyday or alternate days, and a growth scan every 2 weeks. If surveillance results permit, then delivery should be done under steroid coverage by LSCS between 32 and 34 weeks in AEDV and a few weeks earlier in REDV provided no absolute indication for delivery arises in the results of earlier weeks.

If the DV Doppler is abnormal with increased PI or absent or reverses a wave the risk of stillbirth is too high and intensive inpatient monitoring with daily Doppler and twice daily BPP/NST is advised and delivery considered between 26 and 30 weeks under steroid and magnesium sulfate coverage.

MATERNAL CORTICOSTEROIDS

It should be offered to women between 24 + 0 and 33 + 6 weeks who are having a planned preterm birth and can be offered up to 35 + 6 weeks.[17]

MAGNESIUM SULFATE

Should be offered from gestestional age 24 weeks to 33 + 6 days for neuroprotection of the baby, when the delivery is planned or imminent in the next 24 hours. A 4 g intravenous bolus of magnesium sulfate is administered over 15 minutes, followed by an intravenous infusion of 1 g/hour until the birth or for 24 hours (whichever is sooner). If magnesium sulfate is administered 4 hourly monitoring for toxicity should be done. Monitoring should be done for pulse, blood pressure (BP), urine output, and deep tendon reflexes, and respiratory rate.[17]

VAGINAL VERSUS LOWER SEGMENT CESAREAN SECTION

In early-onset FGR, the rate of primary caesarean section is higher.[18,19]

Labor is a stressful process for the fetus and in early-onset FGR, there is always an effort to prolong pregnancy for fetal maturation and bring it as close to term as possible through intensive monitoring. The fetus may already be compromised with certain degrees of hypoxia and acidosis in the process of expectant management and may not be able to withstand further stress of labor.[18,8]

Moreover, the cervix may also not be prepared for induction. Hence, most of the early-onset preterm FGR babies are delivered by cesarean section, Contrary to this, the late-onset FGR fetuses are more mature, acidosis, and hypoxia are unlikely in such cases and can withstand labor trials related to the induction method. Some authors have preferred balloon catheters and other mechanical methods over dinoprostone gel for fewer intrapartum complications and fewer cesarean deliveries.[20]

Continuous FHR monitoring/CTG is recommended during labor. Place of delivery should be well equipped for proper neonatal care as per gestational age.

Examination of the placenta is recommended for placental pathology as per the Consensus Statement of the Amsterdam Placental Workshop.[21]

At all stages, the decision to deliver should be a shared one after making obstetricians, neonatologists, and parents part of the decision-making team.

CONCLUSION

Fetal growth restriction poses a challenge for the treating obstetrician in both timely diagnosis and differentiating it from small for gestational age fetuses. Moreover, the dilemma regarding optimal management is additional challenge.

The main concern in management is stillbirth versus prematurity. Judicious use and interpretation of the monitoring tools with caution and expertise guides a balanced decision. At all stages, the importance of shared decision between parents and obstetrician is the need of the hour.

REFERENCES

1. Fetal Growth Restriction: ACOG Practice Bulletin, Number 227. Obstet Gynecol. 2021;137(2):e16-28.
2. Lees C, Marlow N, Arabin B, Bilardo CM, Brezinka C, Derks JB, et al. Perinatal morbidity and mortality in early-onset fetal growth restriction: cohort outcomes of the trial of randomized umbilical and fetal flow in Europe (TRUFFLE). Ultrasound Obstet Gynecol. 2013;42(4):400-8.
3. Melamed N, Baschat A, Yinon Y, Athanasiadis A, Mecacci F, Figueras F, et al. FIGO (International Federation of Gynecology and Obstetrics) initiative on fetal growth: best practice advice for screening, diagnosis, and management of fetal growth restriction. Int J Gynaecol Obstet. 2021;152(Suppl 1):3-57.
4. Tuffnell DJ, Cartmill RS, Lilford RJ. Fetal movements; factors affecting their perception. Eur J Obstet Gynecol Reprod Biol. 1991;39(3):165-7.
5. Huecker BR, Jamil RT, Thistle J. Fetal movement. In: StatPearls [Internet]. Treasure Island (FL): StatPearls Publishing; 2024.
6. In: Aria F, Bhide AG, Arulkumaran S, Damania K, Daftary SN (Eds). Arias' Practical Guide to High-Risk Pregnancy and Delivery, 5th edition. Gurugram, India: Elsevier; 2019.
7. Caradeux J, Martinez-Portilla RJ, Basuki TR, Kiserud T, Figueras F. Risk of fetal death in growth-restricted fetuses with umbilical and/or ductus venosus absent or reversed end-diastolic velocities before 34 weeks of gestation: a systematic review and meta-analysis. Am J Obstet Gynecol. 2018;218(2S):S774-82.e21.
8. Turan OM, Turan S, Gungor S, Berg C, Moyano D, Gembruch U, et al. Progression of Doppler abnormalities in intrauterine growth restriction. Ultrasound Obstet Gynecol. 2008;32(2):160-7.

9. Bahado-Singh RO, Kovanci E, Jeffres A, Oz U, Deren O, Copel J, et al. The Doppler cerebroplacental ratio and perinatal outcome in intrauterine growth restriction. Am J Obstet Gynecol. 1999;180(3 Pt 1):750-6.
10. Crimmins S, Desai A, Block-Abraham D, Berg C, Gembruch U, Baschat AA. A comparison of Doppler and biophysical findings between liveborn and stillborn growth-restricted fetuses. Am J Obstet Gynecol. 2014;211(6):669.e1-10.
11. Vayssière C, Sentilhes L, Ego A, Bernard C, Cambourieu D, Flamant C, et al. Fetal growth restriction and intra-uterine growth restriction: guidelines for clinical practice from the French College of Gynaecologists and Obstetricians Eur J Obstet Gynecol Reprod Biol. 2015;193:10-8.
12. Nabhan AF, Abdelmoula YA. Amniotic fluid index versus single deepest vertical pocket as a screening test for preventing adverse pregnancy outcome. Cochrane Database Syst Rev. 2008;2008(3):CD006593.
13. Zhang J, Troendle J, Meikle S, Klebanoff MA, Rayburn WF. Isolated oligohydramnios is not associated with adverse perinatal outcomes. BJOG. 2004;111(3):220-5.
14. In: Royal College of Obstetricians and Gynaecologists (Ed). The investigation and the management of the small-for-Gestational-Age. Fetus Green-top Guideline No. 31, 3rd edition. London: RCOG; 2013.
15. Kaur S, Picconi JL, Chadha R, Kruger M, Mari G. Biophysical profile in the treatment of intrauterine growth-restricted fetuses who weigh <1000 g. Am J Obstet Gynecol. 2008;199(3):264.e1-4.
16. Grivell RM, Alfirevic Z, Gyte GM, Devane D. Antenatal cardiotocography for fetal assessment. Cochrane Database Syst Rev. 2015;2015(9):CD007863.
17. National Institute for Health and Care Excellence. National Institute for Health and Care Excellence Guidelines. London: National Institute for Health and Care Excellence (NICE); 2003.
18. Cruz-Lemini M, Crispi F, Van Mieghem T, Pedraza D, Cruz-Martínez R, Acosta-Rojas R, et al. Risk of perinatal death in early-onset intrauterine growth restriction according to gestational age and cardiovascular Doppler indices: a multicenter study. Fetal Diagn Ther. 2012;32(1-2):116-22.
19. Lees CC, Romero R, Stampalija T, Dall'Asta A, DeVore GA, Prefumo F, Frusca T, Visser GHA, Hobbins JC, Baschat AA, Bilardo CM, Galan HL, Campbell S, Maulik D, Figueras F, Lee W, Unterscheider J, Valensise H, Da Silva Costa F, Salomon LJ, Poon LC, Ferrazzi E, Mari G, Rizzo G, Kingdom JC, Kiserud T, Hecher K. Clinical Opinion: The diagnosis and management of suspected fetal growth restriction: an evidence-based approach. Am J Obstet Gynecol. 2022;226(3):366-78. doi: 10.1016/j.ajog.2021.11.1357. Epub 2022 Jan 10. PMID: 35026129; PMCID: PMC9125563.
20. Familiari A, Khalil A, Rizzo G, Odibo A, Vergani P, Buca D, et al. Adverse intrapartum outcome in pregnancies complicated by small for gestational age and late fetal growth restriction undergoing induction of labor with Dinoprostone, Misoprostol or mechanical methods: A systematic review and meta-analysis. Eur J Obstet Gynecol Reprod Biol. 2020;252:455-67.
21. Yaguchi C, Ueda M, Mizuno Y, Fukuchi C, Matsumoto M, Furuta-Isomura N, et al. Association of Placental Pathology with Physical and Neuronal Development of Infants: A Narrative Review and Reclassification of the Literature by the Consensus Statement of the Amsterdam Placental Workshop Group. Nutrients. 2024;16(11):1786.

CHAPTER 16

Breech Delivery

Anupama Bahadur, Sakshi Heda, Ayushi Heda

INTRODUCTION

The approach to delivering a breech is a controversial topic in obstetrics. Fetal presentation, defined as the closest anatomical part of the fetal body to the maternal pelvic inlet, ideally involves the cephalic presentation to minimize risks to both mother and baby. Any presentation other than cephalic is considered a malpresentation, with breech being the most common, accounting for around 80% of cases. It occurs in roughly 3% of fetuses at term, where the buttocks or lower extremities enter the pelvis first in a longitudinal lie. Other malpresentations include shoulder, compound, umbilical cord, face, and brow presentations. While most breech fetuses have normal anatomy, this presentation is linked to an elevated risk of congenital malformations, as well as mild deformities, torticollis, and developmental dysplasia of the hip.

CLASSIFICATION OF BREECH

Breech presentation is categorized as:

- *Frank breech:* In this presentation, both hips are flexed, and both knees are extended, positioning the feet adjacent to the head. It represents the majority, accounting for 50–70% of breech fetuses at term.
- *Complete breech:* Here, both hips and both knees are flexed. This type comprises 5–10% of breech fetuses at term.
- *Incomplete breech:* In this variation, one or both hips lack complete flexion. It constitutes 10–40% of breech fetuses at term. This type can manifest as footling breech (where one leg is extended) or double footling breech (where both legs are extended).

In frank and complete breech presentations, the thighs and trunk simultaneously pass through the birth canal due to the specific positioning of the hips and knees.[1] This alignment facilitates a smoother passage of the shoulders and head during delivery. Conversely, incomplete breech presentation involves one or both hips being unflexed, resulting in a passage of both, thighs and trunk through the birth canal. This smaller fetal diameter increases the risk of complications such as entrapment of the shoulders or head during delivery. Additionally, the smaller diameter provides space for umbilical cord prolapse, further increasing the risk of hypoxic injury.

A study conducted by Jennewein et al., known as the FRABAT study, involving planned vaginal breech deliveries (284 complete or incomplete breech and 884 frank breech), revealed that umbilical cord prolapse was more common in nonfrank breech compared to frank breech presentations, leading to a cesarean birth in a higher percentage of cases in the nonfrank breech group.

PREVALENCE

Breech presentation is observed in approximately 3–5% of pregnancies at term. The frequency of breech decreases as gestational age progresses, with rates possibly reaching as high as 25% before the 28th week of gestation, but by the 32nd week, it decreases to around 7%.[2]

Consequently, prior to reaching full term, breech is commonly considered a temporary occurrence, particularly before the 35th week. Beyond this point, spontaneous reversion to a vertex presentation occurs in fewer than 10% of cases.

Currently, there is a consensus that all expectant mothers without any contraindication should be offered a trial of external cephalic version (ECV). While alternative methods such as acupuncture, mobilization, assuming the knee-elbow position, and others have shown promising outcomes, empirical data supporting their efficacy are limited.[3]

ETIOPATHOGENESIS

The underlying causes of breech presentation are not thoroughly understood, with many obstetricians considering it an incidental occurrence. However, breech presentation tends to be more prevalent in cases where there are accompanying fetal, uterine, or placental abnormalities.

During early pregnancy, the likelihood of breech is more because the smaller fetus can easily rotate within a relatively large volume of amniotic fluid. The reason behind the majority of fetuses assuming a cephalic presentation remains a subject of debate. One hypothesis suggests that a fetus with normal anatomy, activity levels, amniotic fluid volume, and placental positioning tends to adopt a cephalic presentation toward the end of pregnancy, as it provides the most optimal fit within the intrauterine space. However, if any of these variables are abnormal, the likelihood of a breech presentation increases.

Hence, there is a need to evaluate for potential underlying anomalies when a fetal malpresentation is detected at term in a singleton pregnancy as breech is associated with various risk factors.

RISK FACTORS

Multiple factors have been associated with an increased risk for breech presentation, which can be categorized into three main groups:[1]

1. *Maternal:*
   a. Preterm pregnancy
   b. History of breech in a previous pregnancy

   c. Multiparity
   d. Contracted maternal pelvis
   e. Hypothyroidism
   f. Gestational diabetes
   g. Smoking
   h. Extremes of age
2. *Fetal:*
   a. Fetal neurologic deficit
   b. Fetal anomaly (anencephaly, hydrocephaly, sacrococcygeal teratoma, and neck mass)
   c. Short umbilical cord
   d. Extended fetal legs
   e. Crowding from multiple gestation
   f. Macrosomia
   g. Fetal asphyxia
   h. Fetal growth restriction
   i. Female gender
3. *Uteroplacental:*
   a. Extremes of amniotic fluid volume (oligohydramnios and polyhydramnios)
   b. Uterine anomalies (bicornuate and unicornuate uterus and uterine didelphys)
   c. Fibroid
   d. Placental location (placenta previa and cornual placenta)

Risk of recurrence: Data from population-based registries indicate an elevated risk of recurrent breech presentation:

- Following a single pregnancy with breech presentation, the recurrence rate for the subsequent pregnancy is approximately 9%.
- After two consecutive pregnancies featuring breech presentation, the recurrence rate for the subsequent pregnancy rises to approximately 25%.
- In cases of three consecutive pregnancies with breech presentation, the likelihood of recurrence in the next pregnancy can escalate to as high as 40%.

Recurrence is typically attributed to the persistence of fetal, maternal, or placental abnormalities. However, the possibility of a heritable component influencing fetal presentation, which could be inherited from either parent, has been suggested. This speculation is supported by the observation that parents born via breech presentation at term are twice as likely to have firstborn offspring in breech presentation compared to those born in a cephalic presentation.

DIAGNOSIS

Diagnosing a breech presentation involves abdominal examination techniques such as the Leopold maneuvers, in conjunction with per-vaginal examination. Ultrasound confirms the diagnosis.

During the physical examination, using the Leopold maneuvers, the presence of a firm, round, and movable structure at the fundus, along with absence of a palpable presenting part in the upper abdomen above the pubic bone or an engaged breech in the same area, should arouse suspicion of a breech presentation.

In per-vaginal examination, indicators may include the absence of a palpable presenting part, detection of a lower extremity (typically a foot), or identification of the soft tissue of the fetal buttocks if the breech is engaged. Caution is warranted during labor, as the soft tissue of the fetal buttocks may be mistaken for the caput of the fetal vertex.

Any of these findings should trigger suspicion and ultrasound should be performed, which is considered the gold standard for diagnosing fetal malpresentation. Ultrasound facilitates evaluation of fetal presentation, presenting part, and the positioning of the hips and knees (different types of breeches). Additionally, it allows assessment of various other factors including placental location, umbilical cord, amniotic fluid volume, estimated fetal weight, and fetal anatomy review, if not previously conducted. Ultrasonography also enables visualization of fetal or uterine contraindications for vaginal delivery, such as hyperextension of the fetal head or large uterine fibroids. Further advantages of ultrasound include its affordability, accessibility, and minimal adverse effects.[1]

While abdominal X-ray, computed tomography scans, and magnetic resonance imaging can visualize a noncephalic-presenting fetus, they are not recommended for routine clinical use.

ROUTE OF DELIVERY

The discussion surrounding the management of breech delivery, whether through vaginal birth or cesarean section, has become one of the most controversial topics in obstetrics in recent years. Breech birth poses significant challenges due to the persistence of recommendations made over two decades ago, a shortage of adequately experienced and skilled healthcare providers, and the unique clinical circumstances that each woman may face. Discrepancies exist among clinical practice guidelines regarding the management of breech presentation, adding to the complexity of the issue. The primary concern for women diagnosed with a breech presentation is the safety and well-being of their baby, which remains the central focus of modern maternity care. Regardless of the method of delivery—vaginal or cesarean—breech births have been associated with higher rates of morbidity and mortality compared to cephalic births.

Vaginal delivery of a breech presentation is particularly challenging for obstetricians. Despite the global increase in cesarean section rates for breech presentation, vaginal breech births still occur, highlighting the ongoing controversy surrounding this clinical issue.[4]

However, patients and obstetricians should be aware that there is insufficient evidence to conclusively favor cesarean section over assisted vaginal delivery for breech babies, provided that specific criteria are met. Cesarean section poses a greater risk of postpartum morbidity in developed countries and carries significant potential complications, including higher risk of infection, deep vein thrombosis, postpartum hemorrhage, extended hospital stays, anemia, urinary tract infections, wound dehiscence, endometritis, fever, abnormal bleeding, stress urinary incontinence, and increased risks such as abnormal placental implantation and uterine rupture.

Considering the desire of many women for larger families and the rising incidence of repeat cesarean sections due to previous ones, this aspect becomes crucial in the discussion of birthing options for family planning purposes, especially for a primigravida. Therefore, vaginal delivery of a breech baby is a necessary obstetrical skill as approximately 4% of term babies present in the breech position.

Eventually, a woman admitted to the delivery ward with her fetus in breech presentation will expect that a skillful obstetrician will deliver her safely. Unfortunately, at present, most residents lack adequate training in planned vaginal breech delivery. This is the crux of the matter: How proficient are modern obstetricians in performing vaginal breech delivery, and is the expectant mother being provided a fair opportunity to choose the mode of delivery?[5]

There are instances where a woman presents with a breech presentation at the delivery ward, and a cesarean section is not feasible due to medical contraindications, limited facility availability, advanced labor progression, or the patient's refusal to undergo surgery. Consequently, pregnant women with breech-presenting fetuses at or near term are typically offered ECV, as persistent breech presentation often leads to a planned cesarean.

To gather more evidence-based data, the term breech trial (TBT) was conducted in 2000. This trial, the largest randomized controlled trial ever conducted on the subject, compared vaginal breech delivery with planned cesarean. It involved 121 centers across 26 countries and included 2,183 term-pregnant women with fetuses in the breech presentation who were randomized for either planned cesarean or vaginal breech delivery. The primary outcomes assessed were maternal and neonatal mortality and morbidity. The trial was prematurely halted as interim analysis suggested that planned cesarean was superior to vaginal breech delivery in terms of perinatal mortality and morbidity. This single study significantly and universally impacted medical practice, effectively leading to the removal of planned vaginal delivery from labor rooms in the Western world.[6]

In 2006, the PREMODA multicenter study was published, prompting The American College of Obstetricians and Gynecologists to revise their protocols. They concluded that vaginal delivery for breech presentation in single-term pregnancies could be a viable option for appropriately selected pregnant women under the care of experienced healthcare professionals. Consequently, the findings of the TBT came under scrutiny, leading to some national associations incorporating the possibility of vaginal breech delivery into their childbirth care protocols for full-term breech presentation, provided that there are adequately trained personnel at the facility.[7]

Term breech presentation necessitates personalized obstetrical care. In pursuit of a global consensus and shared vision for managing term breech presentation, the optimal approach involves the following steps:

1. Conducting efficient screening for breech presentation at 36–37 weeks of gestation
2. Conducting a comprehensive evaluation of maternal-fetal condition, fetal weight and growth potential, as well as the type (frank, complete, or footling) and mobility of breech presentation. Consideration should also be given to obstetric history and pelvic size/conformation.
3. Organizing a management plan that includes ECV and follow-up during the final weeks, taking into consideration antenatal risk factors. Cases of fetal overgrowth or growth restriction and/or oligohydramnios may necessitate timely cesarean section, and the delivery mode should be reassessed as required based on obstetric conditions (e.g., estimated fetal weight and Bishop score) to facilitate personalized care tailored to each individual's circumstances in the final weeks of pregnancy.

Careful consideration should be given to the expertise of the healthcare team and the availability of necessary clinical skills for performing vaginal breech deliveries when selecting eligible candidates for planned vaginal delivery, regardless of the chosen mode of delivery. Adequate follow-up during the later stages of pregnancy is essential.

Now-a-days, pudendal block anesthesia is being increasingly used as an alternative to neuraxial analgesia in breech deliveries.

Guidelines from the Royal College of Obstetricians and Gynaecologists (RCOG) and International Obstetric Guidelines (IOG) advocate for the training of obstetricians in breech delivery skills. The RCOG has also involved midwives in their peer-review process.

Supraregional centers specializing in breech delivery should be established, and basic simulator training should be provided to residents.

Additionally, a system of standby teams comprising experienced obstetricians should be implemented to offer expertise in planned vaginal delivery.

In a recent prospective observational case series by Bogner et al. involving 41 pregnant women, an analysis was conducted to determine the feasibility and safety of vaginal delivery in the all-fours position compared to vaginal breech delivery and traditional support methods. The study revealed that deliveries in the all-fours position occurred successfully without obstetric intervention in 70.7% of cases (n = 29/41), resulting in a reduced rate of maternal perineal injuries (14.6% vs. 58.5%; p <0.001). However, newborns delivered in the all-fours position exhibited increased antenatal hypoxic stress, indicated by a pH of 7.19 [95% confidence interval (CI): 7.16–7.22] versus a pH of 7.24 (95% CI: 7.21–7.27; p = 0.016). Nevertheless, this did not lead to any clinical consequences for the newborns.[8] **Figures 1 to 3** illustrate breech delivery in all-fours position.

Furthermore, a systematic review and meta-analysis were conducted by Fernandez et al. to evaluate the maternal and fetal risks associated with planned vaginal breech delivery versus cesarean for term breech presentations. The analysis indicated that the relative risk of perinatal mortality was 5.48 (95% CI: 2.61–11.51) times higher in the vaginal delivery group, with relative risks of 4.12 (95% CI: 2.46–6.89) for birth trauma and 3.33 (95% CI: 1.95–5.67) for Apgar scores below 7. Conversely, maternal morbidity

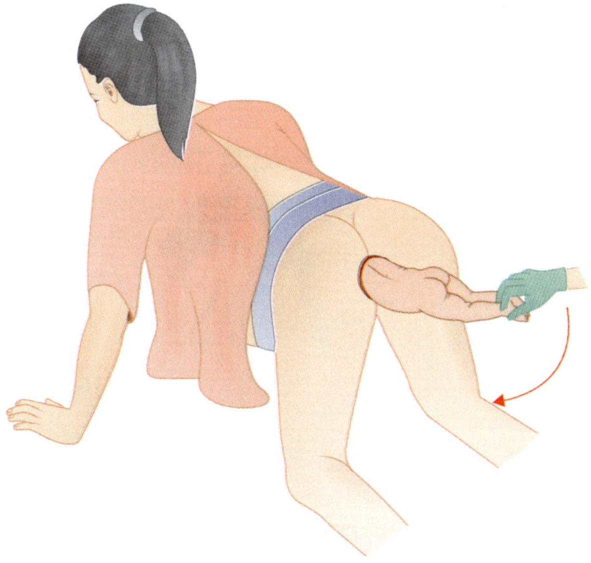

Fig. 1: Grasp both of the child's ankles with the fingers of the hand corresponding to the side of the child's stomach. With a relatively strong pull, we first stretch the child upward and then downward in a wide arc along the inside of the thigh.

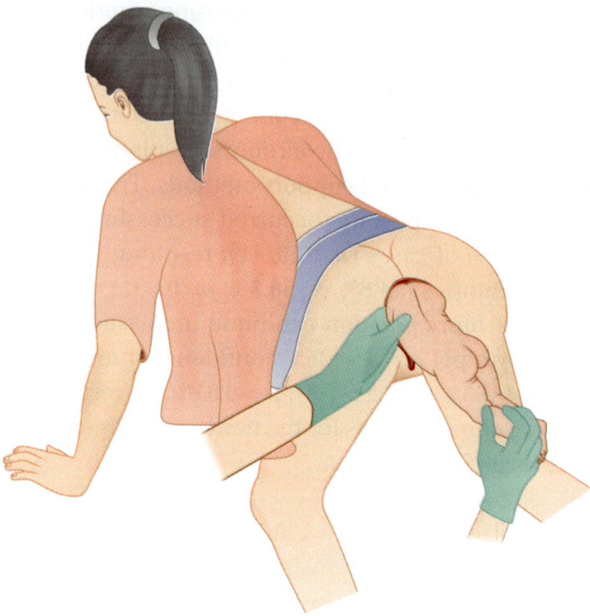

Fig. 2: With our free hand, we now enter the sacral cavity and carefully grasp the child's upper arm.

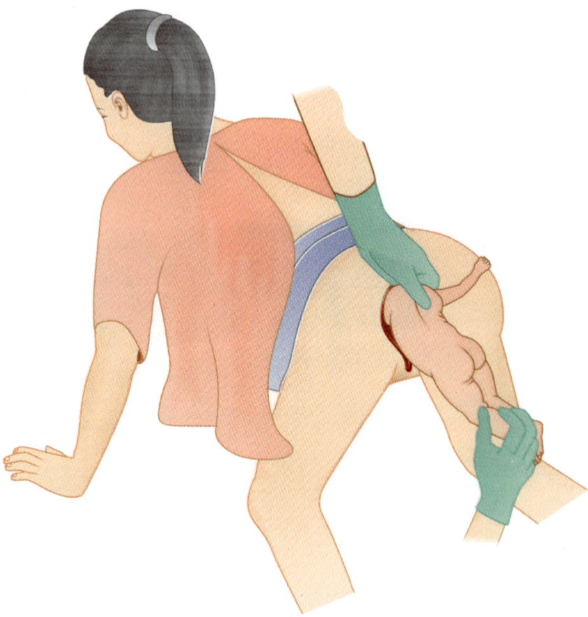

Fig. 3: The upper arm is carefully loosened with the index and middle finger followed by delivery of the head.

showed a relative risk 0.30 (95% CI: 0.13–0.67) times higher in the cesarean group. Although planned vaginal delivery was associated with an increased risk of perinatal mortality, birth trauma, and low Apgar scores, the risk of severe maternal morbidity due to cesarean complications was slightly higher.[9]

Moreover, a Cochrane review conducted by Hofmeyr et al., focusing on planned cesarean section for term breech delivery, concluded that it reduced perinatal and neonatal deaths as well as serious neonatal morbidity, albeit at the expense of a somewhat increased maternal morbidity compared to planned vaginal delivery.[10]

CONCLUSION

The management of breech presentation continues to cause academic and clinical contention globally. One of the most controversial topics in obstetrics in recent years has been the discussion about how to deal with breech delivery, whether vaginal or cesarean. Recent research has highlighted that under specific criteria and with the availability of appropriately skilled and experienced clinicians, vaginal breech delivery can be a safe option. However, the prevalence of cesarean for breech presentation, ranging from 69% to 100%, limits the opportunity for clinicians to acquire and maintain vaginal breech delivery skills in most settings. To address this shortfall, the establishment of specialized breech teams or clinics has been proposed, showing promise in reducing cesarean rates for breech presentation by facilitating increased utilization and success of ECV and providing support to women seeking vaginal breech delivery within predetermined criteria.[11]

The decision-making process for women regarding their preferred mode of birth is influenced by various internal and external factors. Internally, factors such as a woman's personality, past experiences, and personal birth culture play a significant role, while externally, considerations such as time available for decision-making, relationships with partners, family, friends, and interactions with healthcare professionals also shape the decision. Counseling on breech birth is recognized to have a substantial impact on birth mode decision-making. Each pregnancy should be individually assessed for risks, taking into account the woman's preferences and circumstances and aiming to strike a balance between neonatal mortality and maternal morbidity.

REFERENCES

1. Azimirad A. What to do when it is breech? A state-of-the-art review on management of breech presentation. World J Obstet Gynecol. 2023;12(1):1-10.
2. Gray CJ, Shanahan MM. Breech Presentation. In: StatPearls [Internet]. Treasure Island (FL): StatPearls Publishing; 2024.
3. Morris S, Geraghty S, Sundin D. Breech presentation management: a critical review of leading clinical practice guidelines. Women Birth. 2022;35(3):e233-42.

4. Carbillon L, Benbara A, Tigaizin A, Murtada R, Fermaut M, Belmaghni F, et al. Revisiting the management of term breech presentation: a proposal for overcoming some of the controversies. BMC Pregnancy Childbirth. 2020; 20(1):263.
5. Glezerman M. Planned vaginal breech delivery: current status and the need to reconsider. Expert Rev Obstet Gynecol. 2012;7(2):159-66.
6. Lawrence ER, Appiah-Kubi A, Konney TO, Bell SG, Tawiah A, Compton SD. Preferences and perspectives on vaginal breech delivery in Ghana. Intl J Gynecol Obstet. 2021;153(2):307-14.
7. Korb D, Schmitz T, Alexander S, Subtil D, Verspyck E, Deneux-Tharaux C, et al. Association between planned mode of delivery and severe maternal morbidity in women with breech presentations: a secondary analysis of the PREMODA prospective general population study. J Gynecol Obstet Hum Reprod. 2020; 49(2):101662.
8. Bogner G, Strobl M, Schausberger C, Fischer T, Reisenberger K, Jacobs VR. Breech delivery in the all fours position: a prospective observational comparative study with classic assistance. J Perinat Med. 2015;43(6):707-13.
9. Fernández-Carrasco FJ, Cristóbal-Cañadas D, Gómez-Salgado J, Vázquez-Lara JM, Rodríguez-Díaz L, Parrón-Carreño T. Maternal and fetal risks of planned vaginal breech delivery vs. planned caesarean section for term breech birth: a systematic review and meta-analysis. J Glob Health. 2022;12:04055.
10. Hofmeyr GJ, Kulier R, West HM. Expedited versus conservative approaches for vaginal delivery in breech presentation. Cochrane Database Syst Rev. 2015;2015(7):CD000082.
11. Shennan A, Bewley S. How to manage term breech deliveries? BMJ. 2001;323(7307):244-5.

CHAPTER **17**

LGBTQIA+ Issues: The Obstetrician–Gynecologist Perspective

Lila Vyas, Priya Gupta

INTRODUCTION

LGBTQIA+ is an acronym that brings together many different genders and sexual identities that often face marginalization across society. The acronym stands for *Lesbian, Gay, Bisexual, Transgender, Queer, Questioning, Intersex, Asexual,* and *the* + holds space for the expanding and new understanding of different parts of the very diverse gender and sexual identities.

Obstetrician-gynecologists (OB/GYNs) are often the first point of contact between LGBTQ patients and the healthcare system. In 2011, the American College of Obstetricians and Gynecologists (ACOG) published its guidelines for transgender, lesbian, and bisexual individuals.[1] LGBTQ is a vulnerable group with their own reproductive and sexual healthcare needs, which is essential for their overall well-being and health.

Sensitization of healthcare providers: It is important for the healthcare provider to gain experience and training in providing comprehensive and prejudice-free health care to this diverse group of people because of their special needs. So, the approach toward them requires *careful consideration, sensitivity, and multidisciplinary input, gynecologist being an essential member of the team.* LGBTQ patients frequently report having difficulty finding providers who are informed and considerate of their specific needs.

Considerations

- Doctors and clinic staff should be trained to handle them sensitively.
- Clinic staff should be respectful and gender-affirming in their dealing with them.
- They should be addressed by their name, salutations, and especially the pronoun that is congruent with their gender identity.
- They should be treated with the dignity and respect they deserve at every stage of the patient pathway.
- They should treat the patients with utmost confidence.
- Create a nonjudgmental and affirming history-taking practice.
- Pertinent to the OB/GYN, these patient populations require nuanced counseling on sexually transmitted infection (STI) prevention and fertility care.
- *Transgender broken arm syndrome:* A form of medical discrimination faced by transgender and gender diverse (TGD) patients wherein a provider incorrectly assumes that a medical condition results from a

patient's gender identity. It is when healthcare providers assume that all medical issues are a result of a person being trans. The tendency of medical providers to center transness when caring for transgender patients, typically by connecting unrelated medical conditions or symptoms to the transition process, or asking for medical information (e.g., gender confirmation surgery status) that is not relevant to the patient's complaint.

SCOPE OF GYNECOLOGY IN LGBTQIA+ ISSUES

- The LGBTQ community has special needs. Like those assigned females at birth may have problems with STI, abortion, contraception, and polycystic ovarian syndrome.
- Their needs range from hormone therapy to gender-affirming hysterectomies or fertility treatments.
- LGBTQ adolescents are another vulnerable group that has a higher need for contraception. They have more risk of exposure to human immunodeficiency virus (HIV) and STI and less access to needed information.
- LGBTQ individuals have a higher prevalence of certain cancers, chronic diseases, tobacco, and substance abuse.
- A significant number of individuals in this group face violence and mental health issues, which need to be addressed as a part of reproductive health assessment.
- Transgender men who undergo gender affirmation procedures, such as the surgical modification or hormone replacement therapy (HRT), may require gynecological care to monitor treatment effects, which can include vaginal atrophy, decreased fertility, and increased risk of uterine cancer.
- Despite similar gynecological healthcare needs to cisgender women, transgender men experience disproportionately poorer gynecological health outcomes. Research suggests that transgender men face several barriers to accessing gynecological healthcare, including explicit and implicit discrimination, cisnormativity, and fear of mistreatment, leading to distress and avoidance or disengagement with gynecological care systems.

Despite growing recognition and visibility of sexualities that are not heterosexual, research indicates that heteronormativity is a major barrier to relevant gynecological and sexual healthcare for lesbian people.

HORMONE THERAPY

- Transgender hormone therapy, HRT, or gender-affirming hormone therapy (GAHT)
- Sex hormones or other hormonal medications are administered for the purpose of more closely aligning their secondary sexual characteristics with their gender identity.

- Hormone therapy is based on the goal of their treatment whether masculinization or feminization.
- Hormone therapy should only be commenced after the complete psychological evaluation and assessment of the patient for gender dysphoria or gender incongruence.
- Possible benefits and risks of hormonal therapy should be informed.
- Thorough physical examination and concerned blood tests are performed prior to starting treatment.
- Adolescents experiencing gender dysphoria may opt to undergo puberty-suppressing hormone therapy at the onset of puberty, the preferred drug being gonadotropin-releasing hormone (GnRH) analog.
- Feminizing hormone therapy includes medications to suppress testosterone production—estrogens, antiandrogens, and progestogens.
- Masculinizing hormone therapy usually includes testosterone in patient-specific dosing.
- Reproductive gametes cryopreservation should be discussed and considered before initiating hormonal therapy.
- Regular follow-up and monitoring of patients are essential with individualized laboratory monitoring to rule out the risks of hormone therapy, especially in patients with comorbidities.
- Careful assessment of weight gain, acne, break-through uterine bleeding, cardiovascular impairment, and psychiatric symptoms should be done in each follow-up visit.

SEX REASSIGNMENT SURGERIES

- Sex reassignment surgery, also called gender-affirming surgery, is a medical procedure that includes modification of physical sex characteristics and is an important and affirming part of the transition process to align their physical body with their perception of their gender identity.
- This helps them achieve a greater sense of self and reduces their psychological distress.
- Sex reassignment surgery is generally not performed on children under the age of 18 years though in rare cases may be performed on adolescents if healthcare providers agree that there is an unusual benefit of doing so.[2]
- Preexisting health conditions such as diabetes, asthma, and HIV, which can lead to complications with future therapy and pharmacological management, are to be considered before sex reassignment surgeries (SRSs). Typical SRS procedures involve complex medication regimens, including sex hormone therapy, throughout and after surgery.[3]
- In many regions, an individual's pursuit of SRS is either governed/guided, by documents called Standards of Care for the Health of Transgender and

Gender Diverse People (SOC). The most widespread SOC in this field is published and frequently revised by the World Professional Association for Transgender Health (WPATH, formerly the Harry Benjamin International Gender Dysphoria Association or HBIGDA).[4]

- SRS decision/treatment may require a minimum duration of psychological evaluation and living as a member of the target gender full-time, sometimes called the real-life experience (RLE) [sometimes mistakenly referred to as the real-life test (RLT)] before SRSs.
- *Options for SRS for transwomen:* These include genital surgeries such as penectomy (removal of the penis), orchiectomy (removal of the testicles), vaginoplasty (construction of a vagina), vulvoplasty (construction of a vulva), as well as breast augmentation, tracheal shave (reduction of the Adam's apple), facial feminization surgery, and voice feminization surgery.
- *Options for SRS for transmen:* They include chest reconstruction, breast reduction, hysterectomy (removal of the uterus), and oophorectomy (removal of the ovaries). A penis can be constructed through metoidioplasty or phalloplasty and a scrotum through scrotoplasty.[5]

FERTILITY PRESERVATION IN TRANSGENDER

- The fertility preservation counseling should be done prior to gender-affirming treatment (GAT) in all desirous of future fertility with detailed consent.
- Fertility preservation options available are sperm cryopreservation, testicular biopsy, oocyte cryopreservation, embryo cryopreservation, and ovarian tissue cryopreservation.
- Surrogacy is not legal in India for transgender and same-sex couples in recent times.
- Uterine transplantation may be a future option in male-to-female individuals, currently experimental.

CANCER PREVENTION BY SCREENING

An individual's natal and current anatomy, as well as their age and stage with regard to their gender transition, poses difficulties in appropriate cancer screening in these individuals.

Screening is done for breast cancer in both female to male and male to female, whereas screening for endometrial, cervical, and ovarian in female to male is advisable.

SEXUALLY TRANSMITTED DISEASES

- Safe sexual practices are encouraged.

- Patients should be counseled about the risk of transmission of chlamydia, gonorrhea, HIV, hepatitis C, and syphilis.

Despite all efforts, some require an individualized approach with sensitive and special attention to their care and concerns.

CONCLUSION

The LGBTQIA+ community has been ignored in mainstream medicine for a long time. They have special needs and peculiar issues which are unique to their conditions. Obstetrician-gynecologists are a vital part of the medical healthcare professional structure to be able to deal with their problems. A non-judgmental, unbiased approach is essential when dealing with these individuals so that they may feel comfortable with the clinician and may reveal their health issues. Contraception, STI prevention and treatment, gender reassignment surgeries, hormone replacement therapy, cancer prevention, and fertility preservation are some of the most important health issues in this group of individuals which need attention from healthcare professionals. These concepts are well developed in western civilization, and it will be some time before they are approached in a similar fashion in India as well.

REFERENCES

1. ACOG Committee on Health Care for Underserved Women. ACOG Committee Opinion No. 525: Health care for lesbians and bisexual women. Obstet Gynecol. 2012;119(5):1077-80.
2. Rafferty J; Committee on Psychosocial Aspects of Child and Family Health; Committee on Adolescence; Section on Lesbian, Gay, Bisexual, and Transgender Health and Wellness. Ensuring Comprehensive Care and Support for Transgender and Gender-Diverse Children and Adolescents. Pediatrics. 2018;142(4):e20182162.
3. Bishop BM. Pharmacotherapy considerations in the management of transgender patients: a brief review. Pharmacotherapy. 2015;35(12):1130-9.
4. WPATH. (2012). Standard of Care, Version 7. [online] Available from https://www.communitycommons.org/entities/9d0d9ee6-8917-4a9d-bdaa-507da6c20966 [Last accessed September, 2024].
5. OHSU. (2021). Gender-Affirming Surgery: Masculinizing Options. [online] Available from: www.ohsu.edu [Last accessed September, 2024].

CHAPTER 18

Artificial Intelligence in Reproductive Medicine

Rohan Palshetkar, Nandita Palshetkar

INTRODUCTION

Artificial intelligence (AI) is the personification of man-machine partnership. In the present wave of digitalization, the utilization of digital technology in reproductive medicine is not surprising. John McCarthy first used this term in 1955.[1] Artificial intelligence, at its core, is enabling computers to mimic cognitive functions of human mind including learning, analyzing, and problem-solving. Machine with AI lacks human emotions and consciousness. With the increasing use of AI in reproductive medicine, its accuracy is increasing resulting in standardization and greater precision. It helps fertility specialists to individualize patient management in ways much superior to what might be possible by humans alone.

Artificial intelligence has wide applications ranging from automated reasoning (machines completely reasoning automatically) and knowledge representation (diagnosing a medical condition using computers) to automatic planning (automatic cars or autonomous robots). Machine perception is also an important application, wherein computers are capable of interpreting data in fashion similar to humans using their natural senses such as touch, smell, vision, and hearing.

Artificial intelligence allows simultaneous assessment of complex variables critical for human reproduction, both clinical and scientific. It is increasingly being used in our field for analyzing patient characteristics such as age, demographics, and prediction of ovarian reserve as well as in the in vitro fertilization (IVF) and embryology laboratory.

MACHINE LEARNING

Machine learning (ML) is a subgroup of AI, where a machine is meant to learn and adapt to circumstances undergoing self-driven data training **(Fig. 1)**. ML encompasses training a computer program using complex training data sets which uses feeding images describing different features such as shape, color, and texture to make predictions. For example, ML empowers the machine to differentiate between cancerous and noncancerous lesions by taking picture with the camera and using image analysis.

Machine learning focuses on forming automated clinical decision systems to assist practitioners in predicting pregnancy outcomes and planning treatment. ML typically requires reliable databases, providing enormous data

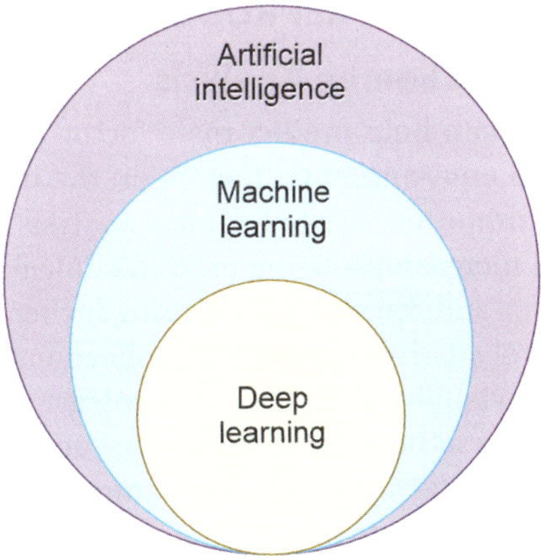

Fig. 1: Machine learning—a subgroup of artificial intelligence.

input for better predictions. In the present era of high-quality data, ML can become an indispensable clinical tool.

Supervised, unsupervised, and reinforcement learning are different approaches of ML.[2] Supervised learning is the most common ML used in reproductive medicine for image analysis and prediction of assisted reproductive technology (ART). This algorithm utilizes labeled data for developing prediction models of a known output. In unsupervised learning, hierarchal clustering is used to determine structure within classes and can be used to predict unknown results. The machines have high energy consumption as they operate at high speed and need a great amount of memory backup, which is possible with cloud computing. Reinforcement learning aims on improvement of the accuracy of algorithms through trial and error.

NEURAL NETWORKS

Artificial neural networks (ANNs) are the most common algorithms for image analysis. It mimics the way human brain works. The neural network is in digital space. Each neuron receives signals from multiple neurons, integrates them, and then fires them in all directions. ML analyzes images using this deep neural network. The computer keeps on refining itself every time, so that next time it analyzes in a faster and better way.[3] The main aim of neural networks is to learn to arrive at an accurate prediction. Neural networks are mainly used in reproductive medicine to predict IVF outcome. For example, Milewski et al. in 2009 created an ANN model for the prediction of adverse pregnancy outcome in IVF cycle. They concluded an excellent result to predict treatment failure with around a 90% probability rate.[4]

APPLICATIONS OF AI IN REPRODUCTIVE MEDICINE

Sperm Selection and Semen Analysis

Artificial intelligence can help predict male factor infertility to study the effect of lifestyle and environmental factors on the quality of semen and fertility rates. The computer-assisted semen analysis (CASA) is no more experimental and is increasingly being used in clinical practice in order to decrease human error and the ease of analyzing higher number of samples in less time. The novel smartphone-based applications can be used for the assessment of sperm viability as well as DNA integrity. Currently, research is ongoing, for selection of best sperm for intracytoplasmic sperm injection (ICSI). A new system is being proposed, which connects the ICSI screen to the Internet, in real time, and then to the AI server, thus guiding the embryologist in identifying the best sperm to immobilize and inject into the oocyte. This application of AI is promising to improve fertilization rates, high-quality embryos, and thus better IVF outcome.

Embryo Grading and Selection

The introduction of automated morphological ranking system for grading embryos is quite beneficial in selecting best embryo prior to transfer. Additionally, the recent use of time-lapse monitoring system in modern IVF centers provides continuous images of the developing embryo and its morphology. Carrasco et al. in 2017 analyzed 800 human embryos with known implantation potential retrospectively with a time-lapse system incubator. They developed a model based on the morphological assessment of D3 embryos, which was helpful in predicting embryos with the least implantation potential.[5] AI can also be used to predict the implantation potential and genetic euploid status of the blastocyst for single embryo transfer. In the future, we will be able to correlate the genetic competence of the embryo with actual visual analysis, and the machine will slowly learn, identify, and guide the embryologist, in selecting the best embryo for transfer.[6] This will obviate the need to perform complex tests such as next-generation sequencing on DNA obtained from the embryo.

Oocyte Evaluation and Selection

The success of ART is largely dependent on oocyte quality. AI has been recently used for the assessment and grading of mature oocytes prior to fertilization or cryopreservation. The AI system exports the images of the oocytes, to the server, which in turn, predicts whether the eggs will yield a good blastocyst and pregnancy, when thawed and fertilized, in the future. The data can also be used to counsel patients undergoing elective egg freezing for fertility preservation. It can help the patient in deciding whether there is an adequate number of good quality eggs, to assure her of a future pregnancy. In case, the good quality eggs are less in number, the patient can decide to undergo an additional cycle of oocyte retrieval and cryopreservation, thus improving her chances of a successful pregnancy, in the future.

Prediction of In Vitro Fertilization Outcome

Fertility specialists can individualize the treatment of subfertile couples and predict ART outcomes using AI-based IVF prediction models. Although the accuracies of different such models have increased to around 85%,[7] further research is needed to apply it in clinical practice.

Embryo Transfer

Artificial intelligence can also guide in performing a perfect embryo transfer, thus improving pregnancy outcome. It can analyze the endometrial lining, thickness, appearance, and the endometrial blood flow. The machine can correlate these images and help us to decide whether the endometrial lining is ideal for transfer or not. If the lining is not appropriate, one can plan a transfer in the next cycle.[8]

Other Uses

Artificial intelligence is also used in administration, medical records keeping, laboratory, and research. Recently, some IVF specialists in USA are utilizing AI to distribute the work in the clinics, so that everyday there is the same number of patients for ovum pick-up. AI can be used for stock-taking, inventory, and quality control, thus improving work efficiency in the embryology laboratories.

DISADVANTAGES AND LIMITATIONS OF AI

- There is a lack of standardization of AI as multiple platforms are being used. The machine should have a balance of good and bad images to guide us correctly. Some laboratories are developing programs, which can eliminate bad data, thus improving results which can be misleading.
- Moreover, the machine must have data based on ethnic diversity, for example, Indian people are different from Caucasian people, hence data from diverse groups is needed. Analysis and interpretation of data in different countries might lead to wrong results. The pooling of information has to be done from multiple data sets, to help us make better predictions. The data sharing implementation and integration of information are important.
- Selection bias from sample collection can lead to poor performance of AI models.
- People are scared that AI may create a lot of job losses with a prediction of 9–47% job loss. The fields involving human-to-human contact will remain in the future, but the fields currently using a lot of automation will be taken over by machines. As the machines are trained, there is a fear that AI will

spell the end of the human race. Stephen Hawking said that "once Man develops artificial intelligence, AI will take off on its own and redesign itself at an ever-increasing rate. Humans, limited by slow biological evolution, will be unable to compete and will be superseded by Machines." However, the opinions of experts within the field of AI are mixed, both concerned and unconcerned by this eventual superhuman capacity. The danger of uncontrolled advance needs to be realized. However, AI will unfold a huge number of possibilities, such as curing disease and better ART outcome.

CONCLUSION

Artificial intelligence is the wave of future which will bring a new era in reproductive medicine. AI will serve practitioners by improving diagnosis and treatment efficiency. The standardization, automation, and precision of IVF driven by AI will provide great benefits to infertile patients and society. Further research is needed in this field by large IVF groups to accumulate the wealth of data needed to achieve sufficient sample size. This will provide broader application of AI with better prediction models.[9] Moreover, AI will not replace fertility specialists and embryologists, rather it will streamline their efforts with better pregnancy outcome.

REFERENCES

1. Wang R, Pan W, Jin L, Li Y, Geng Y, Gao C, et al. Artificial intelligence in reproductive medicine. Reproduction. 2019;158(4):R139-54.
2. Jordan MI, Mitchell TM. Machine learning: trends, perspectives, and prospects. Science. 2015;349:255-60.
3. Niederberger CS, Lipshultz LI, Lamb DJ. A neural network to analyze fertility data. Fertil Steril. 1993;60:324-30.
4. Milewski R, Jamiolkowski J, Milewska Anna J, Domitrz J, Szamatowicz J, Wolczynski S. Prognosis of the IVF ICSI/ET procedure efficiency with the use of artificial neural networks among patients of the Department of Reproduction and Gynecological Endocrinology. Ginekol Pol. 2009;80:900-6.
5. Carrasco B, Arroyo G, Gil Y, Gomez MJ, Rodriguez I, Barri PN, et al. Selecting embryos with the highest implantation potential using data mining and decision tree based on classical embryo morphology and morphokinetics. J Assist Reprod Genet. 2017;34:983-90.
6. Naser M, Mn M, Shehata LH. Artificial intelligence in assisted reproductive technology review. Int J Progress Sci Technol. 2021;25:507-11.
7. Guvenir HA, Misirli G, Dilbaz S, Ozdegirmenci O, Demir B, Dilbaz B. Estimating the chance of success in IVF treatment using a ranking algorithm. Med Biol Eng Comput. 2015;53:911-20.
8. Naser M, Mn M, Shehata LH. Artificial intelligence in assisted reproductive technology review. Int J Progress Sci Technol. 2021;25:507-11.
9. Curchoe CL, Malmsten J, Bormann C, Shafiee H, Farias AF-S, Mendizabal G, et al. Predictive modeling in reproductive medicine: where will the future of artificial intelligence research take us? Fertil Steril. 2020;114(5):934-40.

CHAPTER 19 Sperm Sorting Techniques

Keshav Malhotra, Neharika Malhotra

INTRODUCTION

Sperm sorting, a critical component of assisted reproductive technologies (ARTs), has garnered significant attention in the scientific community due to its potential to enhance fertility outcomes and facilitate the selection of specific genetic traits. This review aims to provide a comprehensive overview of the latest advancements in sperm sorting techniques, their applications, and the challenges that remain to be addressed.

One of the primary methods for sperm sorting is the use of microfluidic technology, which has shown promising results in the manipulation and analysis of individual spermatozoa.[1] These systems offer advantages such as the ability to work with small sample volumes, shorter processing times, and the capacity to manipulate single cells.[1] Sperm sorting techniques have been developed to separate spermatozoa based on their ability to swim through microchannels, cross laminar flows, or swim against fluid flows.[1]

Another approach to sperm sorting involves the assessment of sperm quality parameters, such as deoxyribonucleic acid (DNA) integrity and chromatin condensation.[2] Sperm nuclear chromatin condensation is considered a reliable marker of sperm maturity and has been shown to be associated with the outcome of intracytoplasmic sperm injection (ICSI).[2] The complex journey of spermatozoa from insemination to fertilization involves a sophisticated system that provides sperm storage sites and potentially facilitates selection.[3] A deeper understanding of these intricate processes is crucial for improving the efficiency of conventional reproductive techniques and enabling the development of new ones.[3] The differential roles played by various sperm components, such as the head, neck, midpiece, and tail, in normal fertilization and early embryo development have also been explored.[4] Assisted reproductive technologies have modified our understanding of the prognostic significance of sperm pathologies affecting these structures.[4] The development of medically assisted reproduction has allowed subfertile and infertile couples to achieve pregnancy, with ICSI playing a significant role.[2] However, a notable percentage of ICSI cycles remain unsuccessful, suggesting the need for additional parameters to evaluate sperm quality, such as sperm nuclear chromatin condensation and ploidy.[2]

CHARACTERISTICS OF SPERM AND THE FEMALE REPRODUCTIVE TRACT

Sperm Characteristics

Sperm possess several key characteristics that influence their ability to fertilize an egg. These include:

- *Morphology:* A sperm cell's shape, typically composed of a head, midpiece, and flagellum, is crucial for its function.[5] The head contains the genetic material, the midpiece provides energy, and the flagellum enables movement.
- *Viability:* The percentage of live, functional sperm in a sample is a key factor in fertility.[5]
- *Motility:* Sperm must be able to swim effectively to reach the egg. The length of the sperm and the environment of the female reproductive tract can impact sperm swimming speed.[5]
- *Rheology:* The way sperm flow and interact with fluids in the female reproductive tract is important for their movement toward the egg.[5]
- *Chemotaxis:* Sperm are attracted to chemical signals released by the egg, guiding them toward their target.[5]
- *Thermotaxis:* Sperm can sense and respond to temperature gradients within the female reproductive tract, aiding in their navigation.[5]

Female Reproductive Tract Characteristics

The female reproductive tract also plays a crucial role in sperm transport and selection:

- *Anatomy:* The complex anatomy of the female reproductive tract, including the cervix, uterus, and fallopian tubes, presents both physical and chemical challenges to sperm.[6]
- *Fluid dynamics:* The fluids within the female reproductive tract and muscular contractions influence sperm movement and guide them toward the egg.[6]
- *Sperm selection:* The female reproductive tract actively filters and selects sperm, allowing only a small fraction to reach the egg.[3,6] This selection process is based on various factors, including sperm morphology, motility, and molecular markers.

MICROFLUIDICS FOR SPERM SORTING

Microfluidics has emerged as a promising technology for sperm sorting, offering several advantages over traditional methods.

Advantages of Microfluidics for Sperm Sorting

- *Precise control:* Microfluidic devices allow for precise control over fluid flow and environmental conditions, enabling the creation of complex microenvironments that mimic the female reproductive tract.[5]
- *High throughput:* Microfluidic devices can process large numbers of sperm rapidly, improving the efficiency of sperm sorting (A microfluidic device for separating motile sperm from nonmotile sperm via interstreamline crossings) **(Fig. 1)**.
- *Small sample volumes:* Microfluidics requires only small sample volumes, which is beneficial when dealing with limited sperm samples (A microfluidic device for separating motile sperm from nonmotile sperm via interstreamline crossings) **(Fig. 2)**.
- *Integration with other technologies:* Microfluidic devices can be easily integrated with other technologies, such as imaging and analysis systems, for comprehensive sperm assessment.[1]

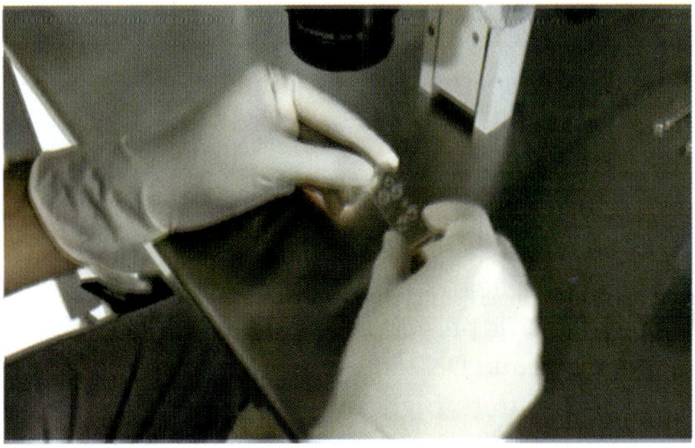

Fig. 1: A microfluidic device for separating motile sperm from nonmotile sperm via interstreamline crossings.

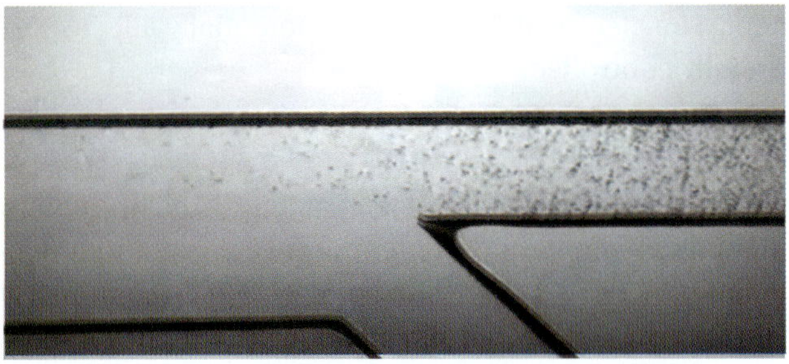

Fig. 2: A microfluidic device for separating motile sperm from nonmotile sperm via interstreamline crossings under a microscope.

Microfluidic Sperm Sorting Techniques

Various microfluidic techniques have been developed for sperm sorting, including:

- *Microchannel-based sorting:* These devices use microchannels with specific geometries to separate motile sperm from non-motile sperm based on their swimming behavior.
- *Dielectrophoresis:* This technique utilizes electric fields to manipulate sperm based on their dielectric properties, allowing for the separation of sperm based on factors, such as size, morphology, and DNA integrity.
- *Chemotaxis-based sorting:* Microfluidic devices can create chemical gradients that mimic those found in the female reproductive tract, attracting and isolating sperm with good chemotactic ability.[5]
- *Thermotaxis-based sorting:* By establishing temperature gradients within microfluidic channels, researchers can isolate sperm with strong thermotactic responses, potentially selecting sperm with higher fertilization potential.[5]

ACTIVE SPERM SORTING TECHNIQUES

Some examples of active sperm-sorting techniques are discussed further.

Dielectrophoresis

- *Mechanism:* Dielectrophoresis (DEP) employs nonuniform electric fields to induce movement in polarizable particles, such as sperm. By carefully designing the electric field, sperm can be trapped, focused, or separated based on their dielectric properties, which are influenced by factors, such as size, morphology, and DNA integrity.
- *Advantages:* DEP offers high selectivity and sensitivity, enabling the isolation of sperm subpopulations with specific characteristics. It also allows for label-free sorting, avoiding potential damage from fluorescent dyes.
- *Limitations:* DEP requires specialized equipment and expertise to implement. The electric fields used can potentially affect sperm viability if not carefully controlled.

Magnetic Activated Cell Sorting

- *Mechanism:* Magnetic activated cell sorting (MACS) involves labeling sperm with magnetic nanoparticles conjugated to antibodies targeting specific surface markers. The labeled sperm is then passed through a magnetic field, which separates them from unlabeled cells.
- *Advantages:* MACS is a well-established technique with high throughput and relatively simple operation. It allows for the selection of sperm based on specific surface markers associated with viability or other desirable traits.

- *Limitations:* MACS requires the identification of suitable surface markers and the availability of specific antibodies. The labeling process might also affect sperm function in some cases.

Microfluidic Flow Cytometry

- *Mechanism:* Microfluidic flow cytometry combines the principles of flow cytometry with microfluidic technology. Sperm are hydrodynamically focused and pass through a detection region where they are illuminated by a laser. Scattered light and fluorescence signals are used to analyze and sort individual sperm based on size, granularity, and the presence of specific markers.
- *Advantages:* Microfluidic flow cytometry offers high-throughput single-cell analysis and sorting capabilities. It allows for multiparametric analysis, enabling the simultaneous assessment of multiple sperm characteristics.
- *Limitations:* This technique requires sophisticated equipment and expertise. The high shear forces within microfluidic channels might potentially damage some sperm.

Advantages of Active Sperm Sorting

- *High specificity:* Active methods allow for the selection of sperm based on specific characteristics, potentially improving the quality of the sorted population.
- *Versatility:* A range of active techniques exists, offering flexibility in targeting different sperm properties.
- *Integration with other technologies:* Active sorting methods can be integrated with other microfluidic components or analysis techniques for comprehensive sperm assessment and manipulation.

Limitations of Active Sperm Sorting

- *Technical complexity:* Active methods often require specialized equipment and expertise compared to passive techniques.
- *Potential sperm damage:* The external forces or stimuli used in active sorting might potentially damage sperm if not carefully controlled.
- *Cost:* Active sorting methods can be more expensive to implement than passive techniques.

PASSIVE SPERM SORTING TECHNIQUES

Passive sperm sorting techniques utilize the inherent properties of sperm and cleverly designed microfluidic structures to separate sperm based on characteristics, such as motility, morphology, and chemotaxis. Unlike active methods, these techniques do not rely on external forces, such as electric fields and magnetic labels.

Common Passive Sperm Sorting Techniques

Microchannel Geometry-based Sorting

- *Mechanism:* These devices use microchannels with specific shapes and dimensions to exploit the natural swimming behavior of sperm. For example:
  - *Straight channels:* Motile sperm swim faster and are more likely to reach the outlet, separating them from less motile counterparts.
  - *Curved or spiral channels:* Sperm with higher motility and better swimming kinematics are more likely to navigate these channels effectively.
  - *Obstacle courses:* Microchannels with pillars or other obstacles challenge sperm, selecting for those with superior motility and navigation skills.
- *Advantages:* Simple design and operation, often requiring less complex fabrication processes.
- *Limitations:* Limited selectivity compared to active methods, as separation primarily relies on motility differences.

Chemotaxis-based Sorting

- *Mechanism:* These devices create chemical gradients within microchannels that mimic the natural chemoattractant signals released by eggs. Sperm with good chemotactic ability will migrate toward the higher concentration of chemoattractant, allowing for their separation.[5]
- *Advantages:* Selects sperm with functional chemotactic machinery, potentially identifying those with higher fertilization capacity.
- *Limitations:* Requires identification and precise control of chemoattractant gradients within the microfluidic device.

Sedimentation-based Sorting

- *Mechanism:* Utilizes gravity to separate sperm based on their density and size. Sperm are introduced into a microfluidic chamber, and over time, larger, denser sperm settle faster, allowing for their isolation.
- *Advantages:* Simple and inexpensive method requiring minimal external equipment.
- *Limitations:* Limited selectivity, as separation is primarily based on size and density, which may not directly correlate with sperm quality.

Interstreamline Crossing

- *Mechanism:* This technique utilizes laminar flow conditions within microfluidic channels. Two or more parallel streams of fluid are established, and sperm are introduced into one stream. Motile sperm can swim across the streamlines into a separate collection channel, while nonmotile sperm remain in the original stream.[7]

- *Advantages:* It can be highly effective in separating motile sperm from a heterogeneous population.
- *Limitations:* It requires precise control over fluid flow rates and channel dimensions to maintain stable laminar flow conditions.

Advantages of Passive Sperm Sorting

- *Gentler on sperm:* It avoids the use of potentially damaging external forces, potentially preserving sperm viability and function.
- *Cost-effective:* It is often simpler and less expensive to implement than active methods, requiring less specialized equipment.
- *Ease of integration:* This can be easily integrated with other microfluidic components or analysis techniques.

Limitations of Passive Sperm Sorting

- *Lower specificity:* Generally, less specific than active methods, as separation relies on inherent sperm properties and may not target specific subpopulations.
- *Throughput:* Throughput can be limited compared to some active methods, especially for techniques, such as sedimentation.

CLINICAL APPLICATIONS OF SPERM SORTING

Sperm sorting, both active and passive, holds significant potential to improve various clinical procedures, particularly in the field of assisted reproductive technology and the treatment of male infertility.

Assisted Reproductive Technologies

- *In vitro fertilization (IVF):* Selecting high-quality sperm for IVF can potentially increase fertilization rates, improve embryo quality, and ultimately lead to higher pregnancy success rates.[8]
- *ICSI:* While ICSI bypasses the need for sperm to penetrate the egg naturally, selecting sperm with normal morphology and DNA integrity using sorting techniques could improve embryo development and reduce the risk of birth defects.

Treatment of Male Infertility

- *Low sperm count:* Sorting techniques can isolate healthy, motile sperm from samples with low sperm counts, increasing the chances of successful fertilization.[8]

- *Poor sperm motility:* By selecting motile sperm, sorting can improve the chances of fertilization, especially in cases where sperm motility is severely compromised.
- *High DNA fragmentation index:* Sperm sorting can isolate sperm with lower DNA fragmentation, potentially improving fertilization rates and reducing the risk of miscarriage or birth defects.

Other Clinical Applications

- *Sperm banking and cryopreservation:* Selecting high-quality sperm before cryopreservation can improve the viability and functionality of sperm after thawing, increasing the success rates of future assisted reproductive technology procedures.
- *Research:* Sperm sorting provides valuable tools for studying sperm physiology, behavior, and the factors affecting male fertility. This knowledge can contribute to the development of new diagnostic and treatment strategies for male infertility.

CHALLENGES AND FUTURE DIRECTIONS

While promising, several challenges remain in translating sperm sorting technologies into widespread clinical practice:

- *Standardization and validation:* Further research are needed to standardize sperm sorting protocols and validate their clinical efficacy across different patient populations.
- *Cost and accessibility:* Some sperm sorting techniques require specialized equipment and expertise, which can be expensive and limit their accessibility in certain clinical settings.
- *Potential sperm damage:* While efforts are made to minimize sperm damage during sorting, further research is needed to optimize protocols and ensure the long-term safety and efficacy of these techniques.

CONCLUSION—SPERM SORTING: A PROMISING FRONTIER IN REPRODUCTIVE MEDICINE

Sperm sorting, encompassing both active and passive techniques, represents a significant advancement in reproductive medicine. By enabling the selection of sperm with desirable characteristics, these technologies hold the potential to revolutionize the treatment of male infertility and enhance the success rates of assisted reproductive technologies.

From microfluidic devices mimicking the natural selection pressures of the female reproductive tract to sophisticated systems utilizing electric fields and magnetic labels, sperm sorting offers a diverse toolkit for isolating sperm based on motility, morphology, DNA integrity, and other crucial factors.

While challenges remain in terms of standardization, cost-effectiveness, and ensuring minimal sperm damage, ongoing research, and technological advancements continue to refine these techniques. As our understanding of sperm biology deepens, we can anticipate even more sophisticated and effective sperm-sorting methods emerging in the future.

The ultimate goal of sperm sorting is to improve the lives of individuals and couples facing infertility, offering them a greater chance of experiencing the joy of parenthood. With continued research and clinical translation, sperm sorting promises to play an increasingly vital role in fulfilling this vision.

REFERENCES

1. Wagenaar BD, Berendsen JTW, Bomer J, Olthuis W, Berg AVD, Segerink LI. Microfluidic single sperm entrapment and analysis. Lab Chip. 2015; 15(5):1294-301.
2. Lazaros L, Vartholomatos G, Pamporaki C, Kosmas IP, Takenaka A, Makrydimas G, et al. Sperm flow cytometric parameters are associated with ICSI outcome. Reprod Biomed Online. 2013;26(6):611-8.
3. Rath D, Schuberth HJ, Coy P, Taylor U. Sperm interactions from insemination to fertilization. Reprod Domest Anim. 2008;43(Suppl 5):2-11.
4. Chemes HE, Sedó CA. Tales of the tail and sperm head aches: changing concepts on the prognostic significance of sperm pathologies affecting the head, neck and tail. Asian J Androl. 2012;14(1):14-23.
5. Huang J, Chen H, Li N, Zhao Y. Emerging microfluidic technologies for sperm sorting. Eng Regen. 2003;4(2):161-9.
6. Vigil P, Valdés-Undurraga I, Del Río J, Serrano FG. The sperm journey to fertilization: a predetermined encounter. Imago Hominis. 2017;24(1):71-82.
7. Cho B, Schuster T, Zhu X, Chang D, Smith GD, Takayama S. A microfluidic device for separating motile sperm from nonmotile sperm via inter-streamline crossings. In: 2nd Annual International IEEE-EMBS Special Topic Conference on Microtechnologies in Medicine and Biology. Madison, WI, USA: Proceedings (Cat. No. 02EX578); 2002. pp. 156-9.
8. Samuel R, Feng H, Jafek A, Despain D, Jenkins T, Gale B. Microfluidic-based sperm sorting and analysis for treatment of male infertility. Transl Androl Urol. 2018;7(Suppl 3):S336-47.

CHAPTER 20

WHO E-MOTIVE Approach

Muralidhar V Pai, Pratik Tambe

INTRODUCTION

Postpartum hemorrhage (PPH) is a life-threatening event which occurs during childbirth. Principally, it is the excessive bleeding that happens after the delivery of the baby. It results in extensive maternal and fetal morbidity. Currently, despite several advances in obstetric care and healthcare delivery, there is one maternal mortality every 6 minutes worldwide. Deaths due to PPH are preventable if optimal care is rendered. The situation is poignant as in some countries, only one in five infants of a mother who has died in childbirth survive longer than the first 4 weeks.[1-3]

The World Health Organization (WHO) and several local and international bodies have given recommendations and guidelines for managing PPH. Unfortunately, there are shortcomings in the implementation of these guidelines as there are multiple barriers and challenges to the same.

CHALLENGES AND HURDLES

One of the primary barriers to implementation is that PPH is not detected early. The CHAMPION (Carbetocin HAeMorrhage PreventION) trial was one of the largest trials ever conducted in this regard that assessed 29,645 patients in 10 different countries. The data from the trial showed that only 26% of women suffering from blood loss between 500 and 600 mL received a uterotonic drug. When blood loss of 1,000–1,100 mL was considered, the number was a respectable 70% of women, but this is still far short of the standard required.[4]

In certain African countries, the primary detection rate of PPH is as low as 2%, which translates into poor implementation of the recommendations from the WHO first-response PPH bundle. It is well known that the estimation of blood loss by naked eye is notoriously inaccurate and results in underestimating the quantum of hemorrhage, which was the guiding principle behind the E-MOTIVE trial.[5,6]

E-MOTIVE TRIAL STUDY DESIGN

The E-MOTIVE trial, which stands for "*Evaluating Medication Options for Treating Postpartum Hemorrhage: Innovative Versus Established Therapies*," aimed to compare the effectiveness of innovative therapies with established treatments for PPH. The trial involved a large number of participants from diverse backgrounds, making the results more representative and applicable to real-world scenarios.

It was a multicentric, cluster randomized trial conducted in multiple countries. The target healthcare delivery providers were secondary-level health facilities in Kenya, Tanzania, Nigeria, South Africa, and Sri Lanka, which were targeted as being most representative of the study population, i.e., mothers at risk for PPH and maternal mortality. It was funded by the Bill and Melinda Gates Foundation; E-MOTIVE ClinicalTrials.gov number NCT04341662.

INTERVENTIONS IMPLEMENTED (FIG. 1)

The E-MOTIVE intervention consists of three elements:

1. A strategy for early detection of PPH, which allows triggering of the "first response" treatment bundle
2. A "first-response" bundle called "MOTIVE", based on the WHO guideline recommendations and consisting of uterine Massage, Oxytocic drugs, Tranexamic acid, IV fluids, and Examination and Escalation
3. An implementation strategy, focusing on simulation-based training, peer-assisted learning, local E-MOTIVE champions, feedback of actionable data to providers, calibrated drape with action line, and MOTIVE emergency kits.

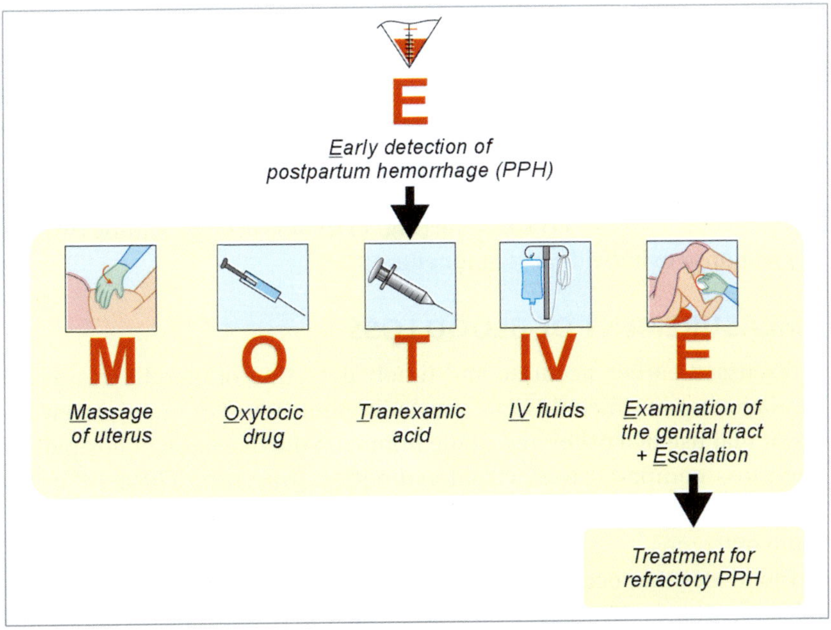

Fig. 1: The E-MOTIVE intervention rationale.[5,6]

Primary Outcomes

Composite of the following three clinical outcomes:

1. Severe PPH defined as blood loss ≥1,000 mL
2. Postpartum laparotomy for bleeding
3. Postpartum maternal death from bleeding

Secondary Outcomes

These were multiple and included laparotomy, use of compression sutures, internal iliac artery ligation, resorting to obstetric hysterectomy, maternal mortality from any cause, primary PPH and the blood loss estimation, use of nonpneumatic antishock garment (NASG), balloon tamponade, blood transfusion, duration of hospital and intensive care unit (ICU) stay, transfer to higher level centers, and neonatal mortality.

RATIONALE FOR "BUNDLE" MANAGEMENT APPROACH

Detection of PPH is most often delayed owing to a multitude of factors. Unlike in other areas of medicine, a sequential approach to administering life-saving interventions results in loss of precious time and maternal mortality. Owing to local practices, restrictions, availability, and economic constraints, some treatment interventions recommended by the WHO may not be used at all.

Tranexamic acid administration—which can be lifesaving—is being used late and only in women who were taken up for surgery, as shown by the survey of healthcare providers in Kenya and Nigeria. Simple, easy-to-implement critical interventions such as uterine massage and intravenous (IV) fluids administration, which can be performed even by paramedical staff, are inconsistently used and may be considered optional by healthcare personnel.

The E-MOTIVE trial aimed to change provider behavior so that there is early detection of PPH and rapid implementation of all recommended interventions of the MOTIVE bundle **(Fig. 1)** *simultaneously*, without waiting for a response to individual components.[5,6]

MEASUREMENT OF BLOOD LOSS

As discussed earlier, accurate and timely detection of blood loss was the foundation upon which this trial was built. A previous Cochrane review has shown that use of a calibrated drape improved the detection of postpartum blood loss compared with visual estimation [*rate ratio (RR):* 1.86; *95% confidence interval (CI):* 1.11–3.11 (high certainty)] but had no clear effect on health outcomes.[7]

Blood loss that occurred after vaginal birth was collected using special collection drapes. Healthcare facilities, which were allocated to the control arm, used noncalibrated drapes while the others, which were allocated to

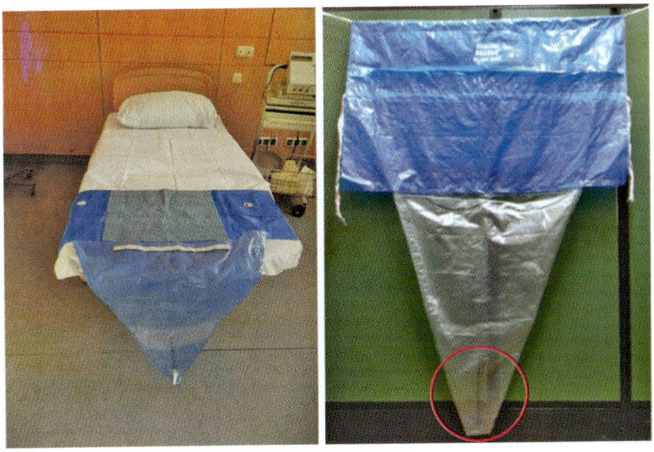

Fig. 2: Calibrated blood collection drapes.

the intervention arm, used calibrated drapes. These calibrated drapes were identical to the noncalibrated drapes. The difference was the measurement lines that were present on the calibrated ones. The drapes were weighed using digital weighing scales following birth and up to the first hour postdelivery. In the event that the bleeding continued, this was extended to 2 hours postdelivery. If excessive blood loss occurred beyond the second hour, a visual estimation of blood loss was performed **(Fig. 2)**.[5,6]

SECONDARY IMPLEMENTATION OUTCOMES

These included:

- The PPH detection rate as diagnosed by a birth attendant
- Adherence to the MOTIVE recommendations.

Adherence to the three core elements of the bundle was necessary: Administration of oxytocic drugs, administration of tranexamic acid (TXA), and IV fluids.

DATA COLLECTION AND AVAILABILITY

Out of 104 secondary level hospitals, finally 80 hospitals underwent randomization into two groups, and data was available from 78 hospitals for analysis (14 in Kenya, 38 in Nigeria, 14 in South Africa, and 12 in Tanzania). A total of 210,132 patients (110,473 in the baseline phase and 99,659 in the implementation phase) gave birth during the trial period. Verified data regarding blood loss was available for 206,455 patients (98% follow-up). The hospital characteristics, patient characteristics, and the availability of essential drugs for PPH (oxytocin and TXA) were similar in the two groups **(Table 1)**.

TABLE 1: E-MOTIVE intervention/protocol specifics.[5,6]

<table>
<tr><th>E</th><th>M</th><th>O</th><th>T</th><th>IV</th><th>E</th></tr>
<tr><th>Early detection and trigger criteria</th><th>Massage of uterus</th><th>Oxytocic drugs</th><th>Tranexamic acid</th><th>IV fluids</th><th>Examination and escalation</th></tr>
<tr><td rowspan="2">• Calibrated drape for the collection of blood, with trigger lines at 300 and 500 mL for the first hour after birth
• Observations (blood loss, blood flow, uterine tone) every 15 minutes documented on the blood-loss monitoring chart
• Blood pressure and pulse monitored once in the first hour postpartum and documented on the blood-loss monitoring chart
• Trigger criteria: Clinical judgment
– Blood loss ≥500 mL
– Blood loss ≥300 mL plus one abnormal observation</td><td>Massage until the uterus has contracted or for 1 minute</td><td>10 IU intravenous (IV) oxytocin injected or diluted in 200–500 mL crystalloid administered over a 10-minute period, plus a maintenance dose of 20 IU IV oxytocin diluted in 1,000 mL saline administered over a 4-hour period (with misoprostol 800 µg if used)</td><td>1 g IV tranexamic acid injected or diluted in 200 mL crystalloid administered over a 10-minute period</td><td>IV fluids in addition to the infusion should be given if clinically indicated for resuscitation and will require a second intravenous access</td><td>• Ensure bladder is empty, evacuate clots, check for tears with an internal examination and placenta for completeness
• Escalate if bleeding does not stop after the first response or the clinician is unable to identify or manage the cause of the bleeding</td></tr>
<tr><td colspan="5">Implementation strategies:
• Audit newsletters: Sharing with all staff monthly rates of detection and bundle use, along with rates of postpartum hemorrhage (PPH), severe PPH, blood transfusion, laparotomy, and death from PPH, and giving feedback at monthly departmental meetings
• Champions: Midwife and doctor to oversee change, troubleshoot, give feedback on audit newsletters, and connect with other champions by means of chats, meetings, and websites for sharing knowledge and lessons learned
• Trolley or carry case: Restocking of all medicines and devices used for the treatment of PPH after every use and completion of a stocking checklist at the start of every shift
• Training: On site, simulation-based, and peer-assisted training, lasting from 90 minutes to an entire workday, facilitated by the us + provider guides, flipcharts, and job aids displayed in labor wards</td></tr>
</table>

OUTCOMES

A primary-outcome event occurred in 794 of 48,678 patients (1.6%) in the intervention group and in 2,139 of 50,044 (4.3%) in the usual-care group (RR 0.40; 95% CI 0.32–0.50; $p < 0.001$).

Postpartum hemorrhage was detected in 93.1% of the patients in the intervention group and in 51.1% of those in the usual-care group (RR 1.58; 95% CI 1.41–1.76), and adherence to the treatment bundle was 91.2% and 19.4%, respectively (RR 4.94; 95% CI 3.88–6.28). The risk of the primary outcome in the intervention group progressively decreased with time after randomization, from a mean of 3.8% during the baseline phase to 1.1% by the last month of the implementation phase.

The median blood loss was 160 mL (range 100–280) in the intervention group and 220 mL (range 120–380) in the usual-care group. PPH (defined as blood loss of ≥500 mL) was diagnosed in 8.5% of the patients in the intervention group and in 16.7% of those in the usual-care group (RR 0.51; 95% CI 0.44–0.60), and severe PPH (defined as blood loss of ≥1,000 mL) in 1.6% and 4.3%, respectively (RR 0.39; 95% CI 0.31–0.49).

There were 17 maternal deaths in the intervention group and 28 deaths in the usual-care group (RR 0.73; 95% CI 0.40–1.31). A total of 12 and 18 of these deaths, respectively, were attributed to postpartum bleeding **(Table 2)**.

HIGHLIGHTS OF THE E-MOTIVE TRIAL

The E-MOTIVE intervention resulted in a *60% lower risk* of the primary outcome—a composite of severe PPH, laparotomy for PPH, or maternal death from severe PPH—after vaginal birth. This benefit was presumably attributable to observed improvements in the detection of PPH and the use of the WHO first-response bundle in the hospitals in the intervention group.

The E-MOTIVE protocol allowed for triggering of the treatment bundle at a blood loss of 300 mL or more if there was an accompanying abnormality in the vital signs or clinical observations. This trigger criterion was commonly used in the hospitals in the intervention group, and this trigger criterion probably underlies the apparent benefit of the intervention for early PPH.

One of the innovative therapies tested in the E-MOTIVE trial was the use of TXA, a medication that helps to prevent blood clots from breaking down. Previous studies had suggested that TXA could be effective in reducing blood loss during childbirth, but the E-MOTIVE trial provided robust evidence to support this claim. The results showed that TXA significantly reduced the need for blood transfusions and other interventions to control bleeding, ultimately improving outcomes for women experiencing PPH.

Another aspect of the E-MOTIVE trial focused on the use of uterine balloon tamponade (UBT), a technique that involves inserting a balloon

TABLE 2: Primary outcomes, key secondary implementation outcomes, and secondary outcomes.[5,6]

Outcome	***Intervention (n = 49,101)***	***Usual care (n = 50,558)***	***Risk or rate ratio (95% CI)***	***Difference (95% CI)***
Primary outcome:				
Composite of severe postpartum hemorrhage, laparotomy for bleeding, or maternal death from bleeding—no/total no (%)	794/48,678 (1.6)	2,139/50,044 (4.3)	0.40 (0.32–0.50)	−2.5 (−3.0 to −2.0)
Key secondary implementation outcomes:				
Detection of postpartum hemorrhage—no/total no (%)	3,870/4,158 (93.1)	4,244/8,299 (51.1)	1.58 (1.41–1.76)	33.3 (26.9–39.8)
Adherence to treatment bundle—no/total no (%)	3,791/4,158 (91.2)	1,623/8,351 (19.4)	4.94 (3.88–6.28)	70.2 (64.6–75.7)
Secondary outcomes:				
Postpartum hemorrhage—no/total no (%)	4,158/48,678 (8.5)	8,351/50,043 (16.7)	0.51 (0.44–0.60)	−8.2 (−9.7 to −6.6)
Severe postpartum hemorrhage—no/total no (%)	786/48,678 (1.6)	2,129/50,043 (4.3)	0.39 (0.31–0.49)	−2.6 (−3.1 to −2.0)
Laparotomy for bleeding—no (%)	12 (<0.1)	7 (<0.1)	1.72 (0.57–5.16)	0.01 (−0.02 to 0.04)
Maternal death—no (%):				
From bleeding	12 (<0.1)	18 (<0.1)	0.80 (0.38–1.68)	−0.01 (−0.03 to 0.02)
From any cause	17 (<0.1)	28 (0.1)	0.73 (0.40–1.31)	−0.02 (−0.04 to 0.01)
Blood transfusion—no (%):				
For any cause	1,074 (2.2)	1,296 (2.6)	0.87 (0.69–1.10)	−0.4 (−0.9 to 0.2)
For bleeding	580 (1.2)	944 (1.9)	0.71 (0.55–0.90)	−0.6 (−1.0 to −0.2)
Blood loss at ≤2 hours postpartum—mL:				
Median interquartile range (IQR)	160 (100–280)	220 (120–380)	—	—
Mean	225 ± 229	318 ± 321	—	−84 (−103 to −64)

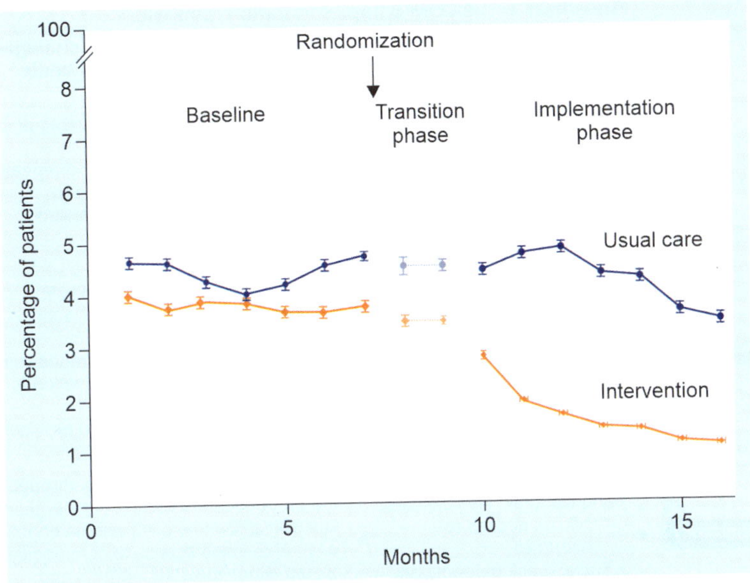

Fig. 3: Incidence of postpartum hemorrhage (PPH).[5,6]

into the uterus to apply pressure and stop bleeding. UBT has been used in the past as a last resort when other treatments fail, but the E-MOTIVE trial explored its effectiveness as a first-line treatment. The findings revealed that UBT was successful in controlling bleeding in a significant number of cases, highlighting its potential as an early intervention for PPH **(Fig. 3)**.

IMPLEMENTATION OF THE CARE BUNDLES

Passive dissemination of guidelines alone may not result in improved quality of care. A robust implementation strategy to identify and tackle known barriers to improve implementation is necessary. The suggested model of behavior change is COM-B, which recognizes that individuals must have Capability, Motivation, and both physical and social Opportunity to perform the behavior(s) of interest. This was one of the key strengths of the E-MOTIVE initiative **(Flowchart 1)**.

CLINICAL SIGNIFICANCE AND IMPLICATIONS FOR PRACTICE

The E-MOTIVE approach compared innovative therapies with established treatments and provided valuable insights into the best approaches for managing PPH. This knowledge can guide healthcare professionals in making evidence-based decisions and ultimately improve outcomes for women worldwide.

Flowchart 1: The COM-B implementation rationale.[5,6]

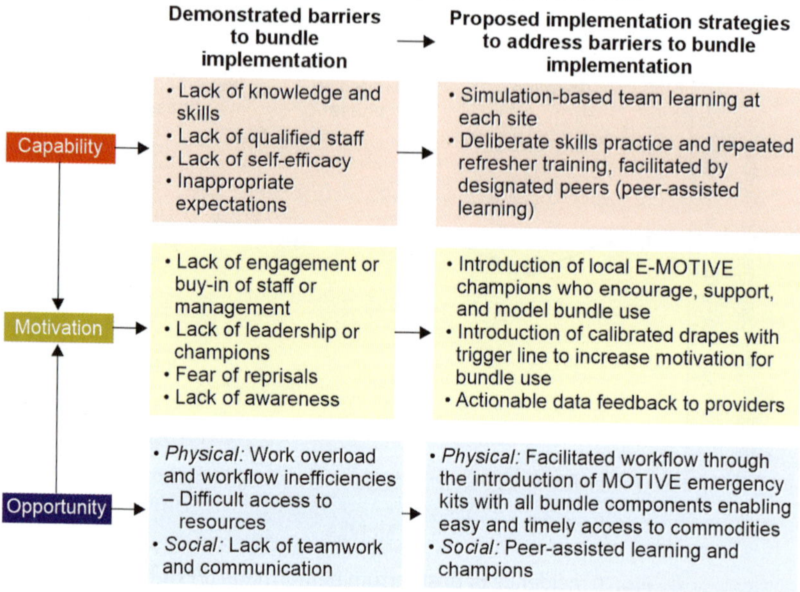

CONCLUSION

The E-MOTIVE approach has brought hope to the field of PPH treatment. This large, international trial showed that the use of a calibrated drape for detection of PPH and a bundle of treatments, supported by a multifaceted implementation strategy, resulted in a substantially lower risk of the primary outcome, a composite of severe PPH, laparotomy for bleeding, or death from bleeding than usual care.

Through its rigorous evaluation of innovative therapies and established treatments, the trial has provided evidence-based insights that can revolutionize the management of PPH. With the introduction of effective interventions such as TXA and UBT, healthcare professionals can now have more tools at their disposal to save lives and ensure the well-being of mothers and their babies. The E-MOTIVE approach serves as a beacon of progress in the fight against PPH, offering a brighter future for women around the world.

REFERENCES

1. Say L, Chou D, Gemmill A, Tunçalp Ö, Moller A-B, Daniels J, et al. Global causes of maternal death: a WHO systematic analysis. Lancet Global Health. 2014;2(6):e323-e33.
2. Family Care International. (2014). A price too high to bear: The costs of maternal mortality to families and communities. [online] Available from https://www.icrw.org/publications/a-price-too-high-to-bear-the-costs-of-maternal-mortality-to-families-and-communities/ [Last accessed September, 2024].

3. World Health Organization. WHO Recommendations for the Prevention and Treatment of Postpartum Haemorrhage. Geneva: World Health Organization; 2012.
4. Widmer M, Piaggio G, Nguyen TMH, Osoti A, Owa OO, Misra S, et al.; WHO CHAMPION Trial Group. Heat-stable carbetocin versus oxytocin to prevent hemorrhage after vaginal birth. N Engl J Med. 2018;379(8):743-52.
5. Gallos I, Devall A, Martin J, Middleton L, Beeson L, Galadanci H, et al. Randomized trial of early detection and treatment of postpartum hemorrhage. N Engl J Med. 2023;389(1):11-21.
6. Bohren MA, Lorencatto F, Coomarasamy A, Althabe F, Devall AJ, Evans C, et al. Formative research to design an implementation strategy for a postpartum hemorrhage initial response treatment bundle (E-MOTIVE): study protocol. Reprod Health. 2021;18(1):149.
7. Diaz V, Abalos E, Carroli G. Methods for blood loss estimation after vaginal birth. Cochrane Database Syst Rev. 2018;9(9):CD010980.

CHAPTER 21

Twin Pregnancy

Vidya Thobbi, Shilpa Nitin Chaudhari

INTRODUCTION

Multiple pregnancies have a substantially higher risk of perinatal morbidity and mortality as well as maternal morbidity. Multiple pregnancies are on the rise as maternal age is increasing. Fertility treatments are responsible for 96% of multiple pregnancies, out of that 36% are of twins and 77% of triplets due to fertility treatments.[1]

INCIDENCE

The peak of higher-order pregnancies has started to decline. The American Society for Reproductive Medicine's guidance for the limits to the number of embryos to be transferred during in vitro fertilization (IVF) cycles aims to promote singleton gestation and reduce the number of multiple pregnancies while maximizing the cumulative live birth rates. Broad guidelines of the American Society of Reproductive Medicine are mentioned in **Table 1**.[2]

THE ASSISTED REPRODUCTIVE TECHNOLOGY (REGULATION) ACT, 2021 INDIA(B)

The Assisted Reproductive Technology (Regulation) Act, 2021 India(b) states that not more than three oocytes or embryos may be placed in the uterus of a woman during the treatment cycle in such manner as may be specified by regulations.[3]

The incidence of monozygotic twinning is constant worldwide at 3.5 per 1,000 live births. This indicates incidence of twin incidents is going to decline in the future, as assisted reproductive technology (ART) recommendations and regulation acts are in favor of the promotion of singleton gestation.

TABLE 1: Guidance on the limits to the number of embryos to transfer.

Regardless of patient's age	Single embryo
<35 years	Single embryo
35–37 years	Single embryo
38–40 years	No more than 3 untested cleavage-stage embryos or 2 blastocysts
41–42 years	No more than 4 untested cleavage-stage embryos or 3 blastocysts

ESTIMATION OF GESTATIONAL AGE

For spontaneous conceptions use the crown-rump length of the longest fetus at 11–13 weeks.[4]

In Vitro Fertilization Conception

In vitro fertilization conception uses the embryonic age from fertilization. If one needs to estimate gestation age after 14 weeks, consider the largest baby in a twin pregnancy to avoid the risk of estimating it from a baby with early growth pathology.

Chorionicity

Chorionicity should be determined between 11 + 0 and 13 + 6 weeks, following points needed to considered:

- Number of placental masses
- Presence of amnion between the sacs with its thickness
- Lambda sign or T sign **(Figs. 1A and B)**

When no first-trimester ultrasound examination has been performed and it is not possible to identify separate placentae and the fetal gender is the same, the pregnancy should be considered monochorionic.

Caution: Cannot apply the above point as Pre-Conception and Pre-Natal Diagnostic Techniques Act (PCPNDT) sex determination prohibition ACT **(Fig. 2)**.[5]

Do not use three-dimensional (3D) ultrasound scans to determine chorionicity and amnionicity.[6]

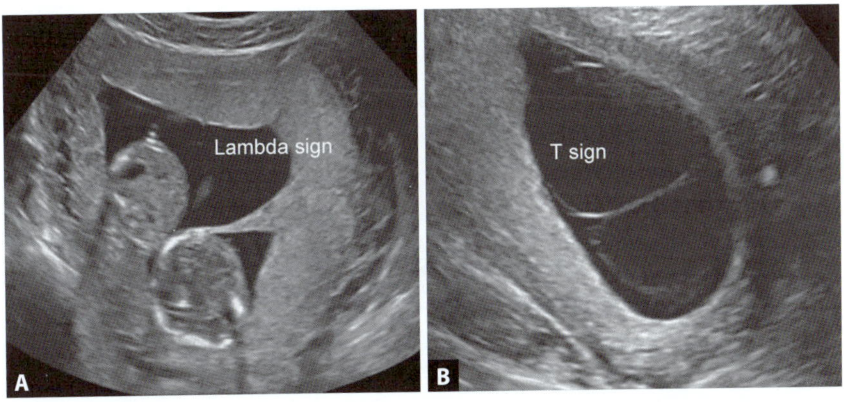

Figs. 1A and B: Sonographic signs for detection of chorionicity.

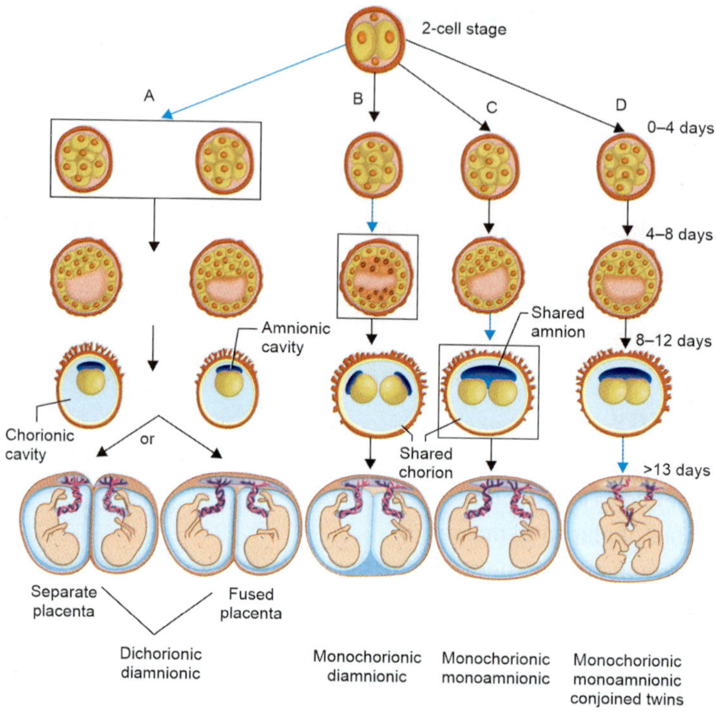

Fig. 2: Types of twins.

PROTOCOL TO FOLLOW-UP IN ANTENATAL PERIOD

Monitoring Scans in Dichorionic Twin Pregnancy (Flowchart 1)

Flowchart 1: Ultrasound evaluation and follow-up.

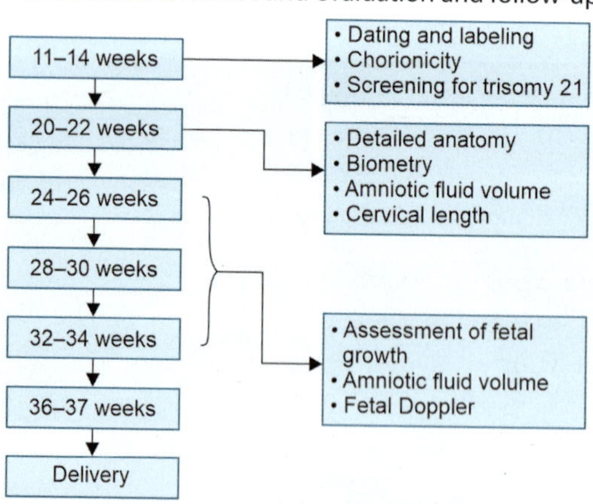

Note: Sonographic evaluation starts at 20 weeks with every 4 weeks follow-up, if complications occur than more frequent follow-up is suggested.[7]

Flowchart 2: Evaluation for monochorionic twin pregnancy.

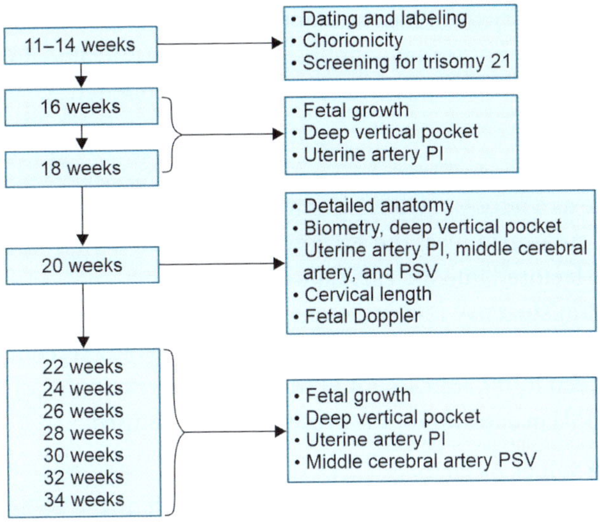

(PI: pulsatility index; PSV: peak systolic velocity)

Monitoring Scans in Monochorionic Twin Pregnancy

Sonographic evaluation starts at 16 weeks with every 2 weeks follow-up, if complications occur then more frequent follow-up are suggested **(Flowchart 2)**.[7]

COMPLICATIONS

In multiple pregnancies, all pregnancy complications are aggravated. The incidence of complications is 83% in twins compared with 25% in singleton.[8]

Fetal Complications Unique in Multiple Gestations as Per Etiological Factors

- *Chronic unbalance transfusion:*
  - Twin-to-twin transfusion
  - Twin anemia-polycythemia sequence
- *Discordant placental territories:* Selective fetal growth restriction (sFGR)
- *Discordant fetal malformation:*
  - Twin reverse arterial perfusion
  - Conjoined twins
- *Acute unidirectional transfusion:* Single intrauterine fetal death

Monochorionic monoamniotic twin pregnancies are at higher risk than singleton pregnancies for aneuploidy.

Due to advanced maternal age in monozygotic pregnancies—both twins are either affected or unaffected.

In *dizygotic pregnancies*, each fetus has an independent aneuploidy risk.[9] Nuchal translucency (NT) measurements are averaged to calculate a single risk estimate for the entire pregnancy using published NT values for singletons.

In dichorionic twins, each fetus is considered separately.

Risk Calculation

- It is done as a fetus-specific risk or a pregnancy-specific risk.
- In both circumstances, the NT and crown-rump length (CRL) of each fetus are factored into the calculation.

Nuchal translucency measurement combined with first-trimester serum markers is the method of choice for prenatal aneuploidy screening in twins. There is a need to do adjustment of the calculated multiples of the normal median (MoM) to account for the presence of two fetuses.

Dividing the values by factors:

- *Beta-human chorionic gonadotrophin (β-hCG)*: 2.023
- Pregnancy-associated plasma protein A (PAPP-A) (MC: 1.78 and DC: 2.19)[10]

Second-trimester screen: High false positive rate. There are increased invasive procedure rates which lead to fetal loss, so it is recommended only when the first-trimester screen is missed.

There is an impact of vanishing twins on screening:

- *If gestational sac empty:* No effect
- *If fetal pole present:* Falsely elevated PAPP-A, inhibin A, and maternal serum alpha-fetoprotein (MSAFP) are seen, so use of NT + maternal age is used to screen.

Prenatal Screening of Twins

Refer **Table 2**.

CONGENITAL ABNORMALITY

Congenital abnormality is more commonly observed in monozygotic gestation. In dichorionic gestation, risk of each fetus same as a singleton, i.e., 2–3%. In monochorionic gestation, the risk is three times higher than in singleton.[9]

Screening for congenital heart disease (CHD) with fetal echocardiography is warranted in all monochorionic twins as the risk of cardiac anomalies is increased 9-fold in monochorionic diamniotic (MCDA) twins and up to 14-fold in cases of twin-to-twin transfusion syndrome (TTTS), above the population, a prevalence of approximately 0.5% is seen.[11]

TABLE 2: Different guidelines for screening of aneuploidy.

RCOG	2016	11–13 + 6-week USG (+serum markers) quadruple test if in the second trimester
ISUOG	2016	First trimester USG (+ maternal age or β-hCG + PAPP-A)
ACOG	2016	11 + 0 to 13 + 6-week USG + maternal age + serum biochemistry
SOGC	2017	11 + 0 to 13 + 6-week USG + maternal age: Acceptable first trimester combined screening combined with nuchal translucency: Less FPR second trimester maternal serum screening if T1 missed (DR: 50–70%, FPR: 10%)
RCOG	2016	11–13 + 6-week USG (+serum markers) quadruple test if in second trimester
NICE	2019	11 + 0 to 13 + 6-week USG (+maternal age)
FIGO	2019	11–13 + 6-week USG (+ maternal age or β-hCG + PAPP-A) quadruple test if in second trimester

(ACOG: American College of Obstetricians and Gynecologists; β-hCG: beta human chorionic gonadotropin; FIGO: International Federation of Gynaecology and Obstetrics; FPR: false positive rate; ISUOG: International Society of Ultrasound in Obstetrics and Gynecology; NICE: National Institute for Health and Care Excellence; PAPP-A: pregnancy-associated plasma protein-A; RCOG: Royal College of Obstetricians and Gynaecologists; SOGC: Society of Obstetricians and Gynaecologists of Canada; USG: ultrasonography)

Selective Fetal Growth Restriction

Selective fetal growth restriction can be classified into three types depending on Doppler study findings **(Figs. 3A to C)**.[12,13]

1. *Type 1:*
   - Growth discordance is positive.
   - Positive end diastolic flow in both fetuses
   - sFGR-90% perinatal survival
2. *Type 2:*
   - Growth discordance is positive.
   - Absent or reversal end diastolic flow in one or both fetuses
   - High risk of IUD (29%), very preterm delivery with risk of neurodevelopmental delay, neurological sequelae in up to 15% of cases if born before 30 weeks
3. *Type 3:*
   - Growth discordance is positive.
   - Cyclical diastolic waveforms—positive followed by absent followed by reversal for several minutes.
   - There is a 10–20% risk of unexpected fetal demise in the smaller twin and a 10–20% risk of neurological injury in the larger twin.

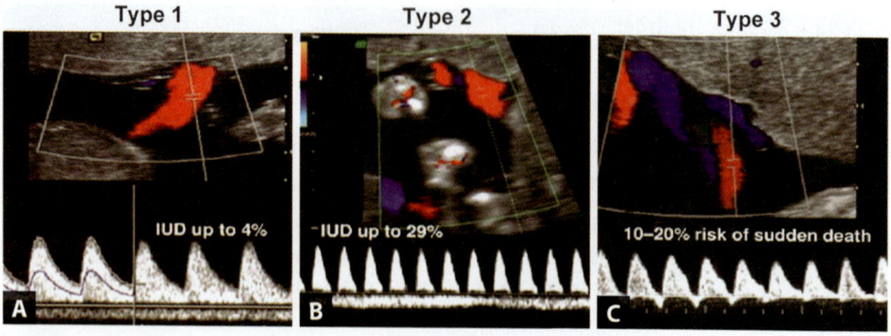

Figs. 3A to C: Doppler findings in different types of sFGR. (IUD: intrauterine device; sFGR: selective fetal growth restriction)

DIAGNOSTIC MONITORING FOR FETAL GROWTH RESTRICTION IN DICHORIONIC TWIN

- Do not use abdominal palpation or symphysis–fundal height measurements to monitor for fetal growth restriction in a dichorionic twin.
- At each ultrasound scan from 24 weeks, offer women with a dichorionic twin diagnostic monitoring for fetal weight discordance using two or more biometric parameters and amniotic fluid levels.
- Continue monitoring for fetal weight discordance at intervals that do not exceed 28 days for women with a dichorionic twin pregnancy.
- Calculate and document estimated fetal weight (EFW) discordance for dichorionic twins using the formula here:[14]

  [(EFW larger fetus – EFW smaller fetus) ÷ EFW larger fetus] × 100

- Increase diagnostic monitoring in the second and third trimesters to at least weekly, and include Doppler assessment of the umbilical artery (UA) flow for each baby, if:
- There is an EFW discordance of 20% or more

And/or,

- The EFW of any of the babies is below the 10th percentile for gestational age. Then the diagnosis is confirmed.

INTRAUTERINE FETAL DEMISE OF ONE TWIN

Fetal Morbidity and Mortality

- In the first trimester, if the death of one twin occurs no effect is observed on surviving twin or mother.
- In the second half of pregnancy, the surviving fetus can be affected by cerebral palsy and cutis aplasia.
- Same-sex twins are at higher risk (2.6%).[15]

- Maternal complications include preterm labor, infection, consumption coagulopathy, and puerperal hemorrhage.
- The rates of fetal demise of the co-twin in monochorionic and dichorionic pregnancies were 15 and 3%, respectively.
- The rates of preterm birth in monochorionic and dichorionic pregnancies were 68 and 54%, respectively.
- The rates of abnormal postnatal cranial imaging in monochorionic and dichorionic pregnancies were 34 and 16%, respectively.
- The rates of neurodevelopmental impairment of the co-twin in monochorionic and dichorionic pregnancies were 26 and 2%, respectively.
- If death of a fetus occurs at <24 weeks' gestation the co-twin is more likely to also die but if it survives, neurologic damage may be less; if death occurs >24 weeks the co-twin is more likely to survive but also more likely to suffer brain damage.
- Ultrasound examination to estimate whether the death of the fetus occurred within the previous 48 hours or earlier (mild generalized edema, ascites, and pleural effusions), and assessment of the survivor for evidence of brain hemorrhage, heart failure, and hyperdynamic circulation with high middle cerebral artery (MCA) peak systolic velocity (PSV). If death is at <48 hours and MCA-PSV is ≥1.5 multiple of the median, then intrauterine blood transfusion should be done and repeat Doppler should be performed after 5–10 hours. If death is at <48 hours and MCA-PSV is <1.5 multiple of the median, then repeat Doppler studies should be done within 24 hours. If death is at >48 hours and there is no evidence of fetal heart failure, then expectant management irrespective of MCA-PSV is indicated.
- *If the fetus survives:* Neurosonography should be carried out in 2 and 4 weeks and magnetic resonance imaging (MRI) at 32 weeks to determine if there is evidence of brain damage. If brain development, fetal growth, and Dopplers are normal there is no need for early delivery.

TWIN REVERSED ARTERIAL PERFUSION (TRAP) (FIG. 4)

- Twin reversed-arterial-perfusion sequence; also known as a cardiac twinning
- *Cause:* Large artery to artery placental shunt (accompanied by vein-to-vein shunt)

Diagnosis

- *Ultrasonography (USG):* Reversed umbilical artery flow in acardiac twin.[16]
- *MRI:*
  - Features of cardiac insufficiency and brain ischemia in pump twin.
  - Detailed morphology of the acardiac twin.

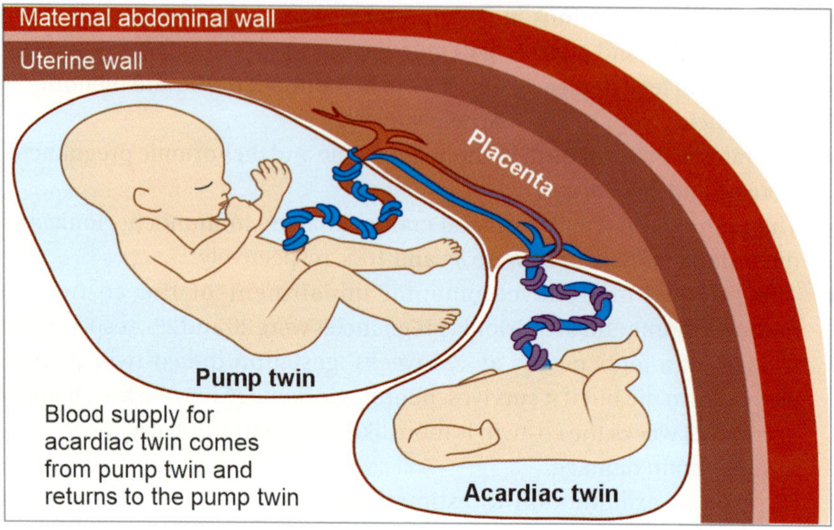

Fig. 4: Diagrammatic representation of twin reversed arterial perfusion (TRAP).

- *<16 weeks:* Spontaneous demise can occur in one-third of the cases. 16 weeks: Umbilical cord bipolar coagulation, radiofrequency ablation[17] without in utero treatment, the perinatal mortality rate for donor twins is 55%. In utero treatment improves survival rates to 80–90%.

Poor Prognostic Factors

- Pump twin hydrops or heart failure
- Pump twin with abnormal Doppler velocimetry
- The calculated weight of the acardiac twin is ≥70% of the weight of the pump twin
- Polyhydramnios
- Monoamniotic pregnancy

TWIN-TO-TWIN TRANSFUSION SYNDROME

- *Prevalence:* 1–3 per 10,000 births
- 5–17% of monochorionic twins
- *Mortality irrespective of period of gestation:* 60–70%
- *Mechanism:* Deep A-V anastomosis

It is a serious progressive disorder.

- Affects 15% of monochorionic pregnancies and 15% of overall fetal mortality in twin pregnancies.

Pathophysiology of Twin-to-Twin Transfusion Syndrome

The pathophysiology of twin-to-twin transfusion syndrome (TTTS) is shown in **Flowchart 3**.

Quintero Classification of the Severity of Twin-to-Twin Transfusion Syndrome[18] (Box 1)

Quintero classification of the severity of TTTS is described in **Box 1**.

Limitations of Quintero Staging

The clinical presentation of a particular case does not always follow an orderly progression of stages. Classic staging is not predictive of recipient survival.[19]

Depends on the severity of the disease.[20]

Treatment Options

- Amnioreduction
- Selective reduction
- Endoscopic laser photocoagulation[21]

Optimal therapy for stage I disease is controversial, and laser ablation or expectant surveillance is an option. Of these techniques, an ablation method may laser individual anastomoses or may ablate the entire vascular equator.

Flowchart 3: Pathophysiology of TTTS.

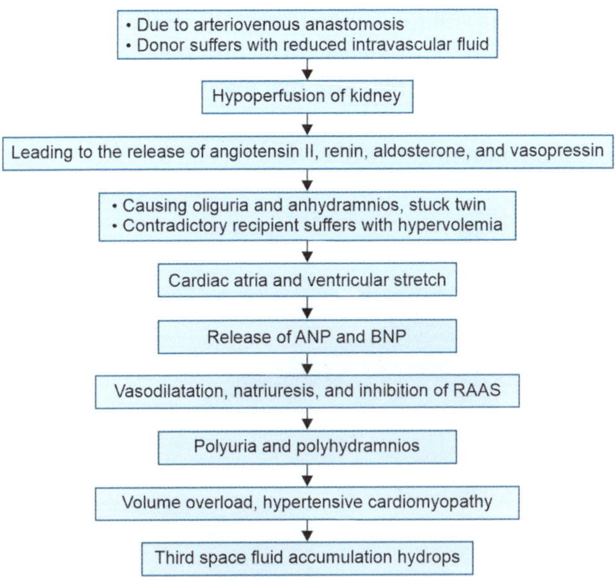

(ANP: atrial natriuretic peptide; BNP: brain natriuretic peptide; RAAS: renin-angiotensin-aldosterone system; TTTS: twin-to-twin transfusion syndrome)

BOX 1: Quintero classification.

- *Stage I:* Oligo-/polysequence and bladder seen in donor twin
  - <2 cm DVP in donor sac and in recipient sac
  - >8 cm DVP in <20 weeks
  - >10 cm DVP in >20 weeks
- *Stage II:* Stage I and donor bladder not seen
- *Stage III:* Stage II and Doppler with one of the following factors:
  - Absent or reversed diastolic flow in the umbilical artery of donor twin
  - Reversed flow in the ductus venosus of donor twin
  - Pulsatile flow in the umbilical vein of recipient twin
- *Stage IV:* Stage III and hydrops
- *Stage V:* Stage III and death of one or both twins

This equator is the border between the twin vasculatures on the chorionic surface. Equatorial ablation, which is referred to as a Solomon technique, reduces the likelihood of TTTS recurrence.

- Septostomy—no longer an accepted method.

Depending on gestation age, management can be advised as follows:[21]

- In type I without TTTS expectant management with close monitoring to define the best time of delivery. If Doppler finding remains normal, then elective cesarean section at 34–35 weeks. There is intact survival of both twins in 95% of cases.
- *Type II without TTTS:* There is a high risk of perinatal death and handicap for both twins if it is ≥26 weeks: the best management is close monitoring and delivery if the ductus venosus end diastolic flow (EDF) becomes negative or reversed. In <26 weeks: The best management is endoscopic laser ablation of communicating placental vessels. Survival of the big baby is 70%, and of the small baby depends on ductus venosus EDF: 40% if positive and 10% if negative or reversed **(Fig. 5)**.

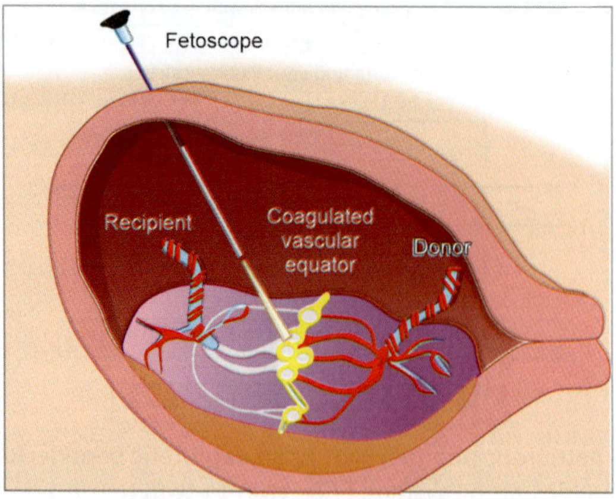

Fig. 5: Laser ablation in twin-to-twin transfusion syndrome (TTTS).

- Risk of neonatal cerebral lesions primarily depends on gestational age at delivery and varies from 20% for birth at <26 weeks to 5% for birth at ≥32 weeks.
- An alternative management is cord occlusion of the small fetus; the survival of the large twin is 90%.
- In types I and II with TTTS endoscopic laser ablation of communicating placental vessels is advocated.
- In type III sudden unexpected death could occur in 20–30% of cases. Laser surgery may be impossible, and the best management is close monitoring and delivery on the basis of ductus venosus EDF in the small fetus. If the ductus venosus EDF is positive elective delivery should be by cesarean section at 32 weeks' gestation.
- There is a 20% risk of neonatal cerebral lesions, and the risk is greater in the larger than small fetus.
  - USG for post-laser fetal surveillance
  - USG weekly for 2 weeks for MCA-PSV and resolution
  - USG 2 weekly after clinical resolution
- Demonstration of bladder filling and increasing amniotic fluid of donor implies TTTS resolution.
  - *Delivery:* 34 weeks (persisting abnormalities)—37 weeks (resolved TTTS).

TWIN ANEMIA-POLYCYTHEMIA SEQUENCE

- A chronic form of fetofetal transfusion in monochorionic twins, characterized by large hemoglobin (Hb) difference at birth
- *Spontaneous TAPS:* 1–6%.
- *Iatrogenic (post-laser) TAPS:* 2–13%

Pathophysiology of Twin Anemia-Polycythemia Sequence

In this condition, there are very small AV unidirectional unbalanced anastomoses seen with less number of anastomoses. There is slow passage of red cells from donor to recipient leading to the donor twin being anemic one and the recipient twin to polycythemic.

Staging of Twin Anemia-Polycythemia Sequence[22]

Antenatal

- *Stage 1:* MCA-PSV >1.5 MoM in the donor and MCA-PSV <1.0 MoM in the recipient without other signs of fetal compromise.
- *Stage 2:* MCA-PSV >1.7 MoM in the donor and MCA-PSV <0.8 MoM in the recipient without other signs of fetal compromise.
- *Stage 3:* As stage 1 or 2 with cardiac compromise of donor.

- *Stage 4:* Hydrops of donor.
- *Stage 5:* Intrauterine demise of one or both fetuses preceded by TAPS.

Postnatal

- Stage 1 intertwin Hb difference >8.0 g/dL
- Stage 1 intertwin Hb difference >11.0 g/dL
- Stage 1 intertwin Hb difference >14.0 g/dL
- Stage 1 intertwin Hb difference >17.0 g/dL
- Stage 1 intertwin Hb difference >20.0 g/dL

Twin-to-Twin Transfusion Syndrome vs. Twin Anemia-Polycythemia Sequence vs. Fetal Growth Restriction (Table 3)

TABLE 3: Differences between TTTS, TAPS, sFGR.

Ultrasound finding	***TTTS***	***TAPS***	***sFGR***
Fluid discordance	+++++ Oligohydramnios in one sac and polyhydramnios in the other sac	–	++ Oligohydramnios in the sac of the intrauterine growth-restricted twin, normal AF in AGA twin
Growth discordance (>25%)	++ 50% will have EFW <10th percentile	+	+++++ 100% will have EFW <10th percentile
MCA Doppler discordance (>1.5 MoM in donor/anemic and <0.8 MoM in recipient/plethoric)	++	+++++	+
Fetal bladder discordance	Small donor bladder and/or enlarged recipient bladder	–	–
DV abnormalities	+++++	++	++
Fetal hydrops	+++++	+	–
Placental appearance: Donor side hyperechoic and thickened, recipient side (normal)	++	+++++	–

(AF: amniotic fluid; AGA: appropriate-for-gestational-age; DV: ductus venosus; EFW: estimated fetal weight; MCA: middle cerebral artery; sFGR: selective fetal growth restriction; TTTS: twin-to-twin transfusion syndrome; TAPS: twin anemia–polycythemia sequence)

PRETERM BIRTH

Screening for Preterm Birth

Pregnant woman and their family members need to explain a higher risk of spontaneous preterm birth than women or pregnant people with a singleton pregnancy. They also need to explain that this risk is further increased if they have other risk factors, such as a spontaneous preterm birth in a previous pregnancy or they are found to have a short cervix on cervical length screening.[6]

There is no role of:

- Fetal fibronectin testing alone to predict the risk of spontaneous preterm birth in twin pregnancy.
- Use of home uterine activity monitoring to predict the risk of spontaneous preterm birth in twin pregnancy.

Preventing Preterm Birth

- Offers a single cervical length scan between 16 and 20 weeks to a pregnant woman with a twin pregnancy.
- There is a role of treatment with progesterone if a cervical length scan shows a short cervix (25 mm or less) in reducing the risk of preterm birth.
- Offer progesterone 200 mg vaginal capsules once a day at bedtime to women with a twin pregnancy and a cervical length of 25 mm or less. Continue treatment until 34 weeks (or birth if sooner).
- If a cervical length of 25 mm or less is found incidentally on a scan conducted between 20 and 24 weeks, offer progesterone 200 mg vaginal capsules once a day at bedtime. Continue treatment until 34 weeks (or birth if sooner).
- Do not offer intramuscular progesterone to prevent spontaneous preterm birth in women with a twin pregnancy.
- Do not offer the following interventions (alone or in combination) routinely to prevent spontaneous preterm birth in women or pregnant women with a twin pregnancy.[6]
  - Arabin pessary
  - Bed rest
  - Cervical cerclage
  - Oral tocolytics

CORTICOSTEROIDS

- There are benefits of targeted corticosteroids in twin gestation, as there is a risk of preterm birth.
- There is no benefit in using untargeted administration of corticosteroids.[6]

TIME FOR DELIVERY

- Uncomplicated dichorionic diamniotic: deliver at 37 + 0.
- Uncomplicated monochorionic/diamniotic twins at 36 + 0 weeks of gestation or soon thereafter and by 36 + 6 weeks are advised (the risks of unanticipated stillbirth with expectant management and the risks of neonatal mortality and morbidity with delivery, which is different for monochorionic versus dichorionic twins).
- The American College of Obstetricians and Gynecologists (ACOG) and Society for Maternal-Fetal Medicine (SMFM) guidelines recommend delivery at 34 + 0 to 37 + 6 weeks and the North American Fetal Therapy Network, recommends delivery at 36 + 0 to 37 + 6 weeks.
- Uncomplicated monochorionic monoamniotic should deliver at 32 + 0 and 33 + 6 weeks.
- In a complicated twin an individual assessment to determine the timing of planned birth in women is required.[23]

MODE OF DELIVERY

- *Both twins in a cephalic presentation:* Vaginal delivery
- *Presenting twin noncephalic and nonpresenting twin cephalic or noncephalic:* Cesarean delivery
- Presenting twin cephalic and nonpresenting twin noncephalic
- *Gestation age <28 weeks or EFW of nonpresenting twin is <1,500 g:* Cesarean delivery
- If EFW of nonpresenting twin is >20 % of presenting twin, then vaginal delivery of presenting twin and external cephalic version for nonpresenting twin is recommended.
- If EFW of nonpresenting twin is >20% of presenting twin, then vaginal delivery of presenting twin and breech extraction of nonpresenting twin is recommended.
- Offer an individualized assessment of the mode of birth to women in suspected, diagnosed, or established preterm labor before 26 weeks. Take into account the risks of cesarean section and the chance of survival of the babies.[23]
- In monochorionic monoamniotic cesarean section to be done in women with a monochorionic monoamniotic twin pregnancy:
  - At the time of planned birth (between 32 + 0 and 33 + 6 weeks)
    Or
  - After any complication is diagnosed in her pregnancy requiring earlier delivery.
    Or
  - If she is in established preterm labor, and gestational age suggests there is a reasonable chance of survival of the babies.

- *Decision to deliver the second twin after the birth of the first twin:*
  - Confirmation of presentation of second twin done if it is cephalic monitor fetal heart sound (FHS), monitor uterine contractions, if require augmentation with oxytocin done and after descent of presenting part rupture of membrane done. If FHS are abnormal or arrest of descent occurs cesarean delivery is opted.
  - If the second twin in the breech presentation if consent is given by the patient for breech extraction or an external cephalic version is given, then that procedure is opted.

CONCLUSION

Multifetal gestations and twin pregnancies are more common today owing to iatrogenic causes. Post-ART twin pregnancies carry a higher risk of complications during all trimesters of pregnancy. Close surveillance and consultation with a fetal medicine expert with a multidisciplinary team approach is of paramount importance to ensure good outcomes in these patients. Fetal growth restriction in one or both twins, TRAP and twin-to-twin transfusion syndrome are all unique issues which require expert management in tertiary care with an experienced team of clinicians to ensure timely delivery and minimize perinatal morbidity and mortality.

REFERENCES

1. Blondel B, Kogan MD, Alexander GR, Dattani N, Kramer MS, Macfarlane A, et al. The impact of the increasing number of multiple births on the rates of preterm birth and low birthweight: an international study. Am J Public Health. 2002;92(8):1323-30.
2. Practice Committee of the American Society for Reproductive Medicine and the Practice Committee for the Society for Assisted Reproductive Technologies. Guidance on the limits to the number of embryos to transfer: a committee opinion. Fertil Steril. 2021;116(3):651-54.
3. DeYoung TH, Stortz SK, Riffenburgh RH, Wren GM, Spitzer TL, Lutgendorf MA, et al Establishing the most accurate due date in dichorionic twin gestations by first and second trimester ultrasound. J Ultrasound Med. 2021;40(11):2319-27
4. Ministries/Departments in the Government of India. The assisted reproductive technology (regulation) act, 2021 ACT NO. 42 OF 2021. [Online] Available from https://www.indiacode.nic.in/bitstream/123456789/17031/1/A2021-42%20.pdf [Lst accessed September, 2024].
5. Salomon LJ, Alfirevic Z, Berghella V, Bilardo CM, Chalouhi GE, Da Silva Costa F, et al. ISUOG Practice Guidelines (updated): performance of the routine mid-trimester fetal ultrasound scan. Ultrasound Obstet Gynecol. 2022;59(6):840-56.
6. National Institute for Health and Care Excellence. (2024). Twin and triplet pregnancy. [Online] Available from www.nice.org.uk/guidance/ng137 [Last accessed September, 2024].
7. FIGO Working Group on Good Clinical Practice in Maternal–Fetal Medicine. Good clinical practice advice: Management of twin pregnancy. Int J Gynecol Obstet. 2019;144(3):330-7.

8. American College of Obstetricians and Gynecologists. ACOG educational bulletin. Special problems of multiple gestation. Number 253, November 1998 (Replaces Number 131, August 1989). American College of Obstetricians and Gynecologists Int J Gynaecol Obstet. 1999;64(3):323-33.
9. Mei-Dan E, Jain V, Melamed N, Lim KI, Aviram A, Ryan G, et al. Guideline No. 428: Management of Dichorionic Twin Pregnancies. J Obstet Gynaecol Can. 2022;44(7)819-34.
10. Sparks TN, Norton ME, Flessel M, Goldman S, Currier RJ. Observed rate of Down syndrome in twin pregnancies. Obstet Gynecol. 2016;128(5):1127-33.
11. Gijtenbeek M, Shirzada MR, Ten Harkel ADJ, Oepkes D, C Haak M. Congenital heart defects in monochorionic twins: a systematic review and meta-analysis. J Clin Med. 2019;8(6):902.
12. Gratacós E, Lewi L, Muñoz B, Acosta-Rojas R, Hernandez-Andrade E, Martinez JM, et al. A classification system for selective intrauterine growth restriction in monochorionic pregnancies according to umbilical artery Doppler flow in the smaller twin. Ultrasound Obstet Gynecol. 2007;30(1):28-34.
13. Khalil A, Rodgers M, Baschat A, Bhide A, Gratacos E, Hecher K, et al. ISUOG Practice Guidelines: role of ultrasound in twin pregnancy. Ultrasound Obstet. Gynecol. 2016;47(2):247-63.
14. Breathnach FM, McAuliffe FM, Geary M, Daly S, Higgins JR, Dornan J, et al. Perinatal Ireland Research Consortium. Definition of intertwin birth weight discordance. Obstet Gynecol. 2011;118(1):94-103.
15. Rydhstroem H. Discordant birthweight and late fetal death in like-sexed and unlike-sexed twin pairs: a population-based study. Br J Obstet Gynecol. 1994;101(9):765-9.
16. Billah KL Shah K, Odwin C. Ultrasonographic diagnosis and management of acardiac acephalus twin pregnancy. Med Ultrasound. 1984;8:108-10.
17. Tsoa K, Feldstein VA, Albanase CT, Sandberg PL, Lee H, Harrison MR, et al. Selective reduction of acardiac twin by radiofrequency ablation. Am J Obstet Gynecol. 2002;187(3):635-40.
18. Quintero RA, Morales WJ, Allen MH, Bornick PW, Johnson PK, Kruger M. Staging of twin-twin transfusion syndrome. J Perinatol. 1999;19(8 Pt 1):550-5.
19. Taylor MJ, Govender L, Jolly M, Wee L, Fisk NM. Validation of the Quintero staging system for twin-twin transfusion syndrome. Obstet Gynecol. 2002;100(6):1257-65.
20. Rossi AC, D'Addario VC. Diagnosis and Management of Twin-Twin Transfusion Syndrome. Donald School Journal of Ultrasound in Obstetrics and Gynecology, July-September 2012;6(3):286-9.
21. Sileo FG, D'antonio F, Benlioglu C, Bhide A, Khalil A. Perinatal outcomes of twin pregnancies complicated by late twin-twin transfusion syndrome: a systematic review and meta-analysis. Acta Obstet Gynecol Scand. 2021;100(5):832-42.
22. Tollenaar LSA, Slaghekke F, Lewi L, Ville Y, Lanna M, Weingertner A, et al. Treatment and outcome of 370 cases with spontaneous or post-laser twin anemia-polycythemia sequence managed in 17 fetal therapy centers. Ultrasound Obstet Gynecol. 2020;56(3):378-87.
23. Cheong-See F, Schuit E, Arroyo-Manzano D, Khalil A, Barrett J, Joseph KS, et al. Prospective risk of stillbirth and neonatal complications in twin pregnancies: systematic review and meta-analysis. BMJ. 2016;354:i4353.

CHAPTER 22

Adolescent Mental Health Issues

Roza Olyai, Manila Kaushal

INTRODUCTION

Adolescence is a critical period of development marked by significant physical, emotional, and social changes. Adolescent girls face unique mental health challenges influenced by biological, psychological, and sociocultural factors. This chapter delves into the complexities of mental health issues among adolescent girls, exploring contributing factors, common disorders, and strategies for support and intervention.

COMMON MENTAL HEALTH ISSUES AMONG ADOLESCENT GIRLS

Common mental health issues include the following:

- *Depression:* Adolescent girls are at higher risk of depression than boys, experiencing persistent feelings of sadness, hopelessness, and worthlessness that interfere with daily functioning and quality of life.[1] It presents in form change in sleep and appetite and loss of interest.
- *Anxiety disorders:* Generalized anxiety disorder, social anxiety disorder, and panic disorder are prevalent among adolescent girls, leading to excessive worry, fear, and avoidance behaviors.
- *Eating disorders:* Conditions such as anorexia nervosa, bulimia nervosa, and binge-eating disorder disproportionately affect adolescent girls, driven by societal pressures related to body image, dieting, and perfectionism.[2]
- *Self-harm:* Adolescent girls may engage in self-harming behaviors such as cutting, scratching, or burning as maladaptive coping mechanisms for emotional distress, trauma, or low self-esteem.
- *Suicidal ideation and behavior:* Adolescent girls are at increased risk of suicidal ideation and suicide attempts, often linked to untreated mental health disorders, interpersonal conflicts, or experiences of abuse and trauma.[2]
- *Attention-deficit/hyperactivity disorder (ADHD):* Although ADHD is more commonly diagnosed in boys, it can also affect adolescent girls, leading to difficulties with attention, impulsivity, and hyperactivity.
- *Post-traumatic stress disorder (PTSD):* Adolescent girls may develop PTSD following exposure to traumatic events such as abuse, violence, or natural disasters, experiencing symptoms such as flashbacks, nightmares, and hypervigilance.

- *Substance use disorders:* Adolescent girls may engage in substance abuse as a way to cope with stress, anxiety, or trauma, leading to addiction and negative consequences for their mental and physical health.
- *Bipolar disorder:* It involves extreme mood swings from highs (mania) to lows (depression).
- *Body dysmorphic disorder (BDD):* BDD is characterized by obsessive preoccupation with perceived flaws in appearance, leading to distress and impaired functioning. Adolescent girls may excessively focus on their appearance, leading to low self-esteem and social withdrawal.
- *Adjustment disorders:* Adolescent girls may experience adjustment disorders in response to significant life changes or stressors such as moving to a new school, parental divorce, or the loss of a loved one, leading to emotional distress and impaired functioning.

These conditions can vary in severity and require professional intervention and support groups.

CONTRIBUTING FACTORS TO MENTAL HEALTH ISSUES AMONG ADOLESCENT GIRLS

Following are the contributing factors to mental health issues:

- *Biological factors:* Genetic predisposition and hormonal fluctuations during puberty and adolescence can impact mood regulation and increase vulnerability to mental health disorders such as depression and anxiety.
- *Psychosocial factors:* Gender norms, societal expectations, peer relationships, and family dynamics influence adolescent girls' sense of identity, self-esteem, and coping mechanisms, shaping their mental health outcomes.[3]
- *Trauma and adversity:* Experiences of trauma, abuse, bullying, or discrimination can have profound and long-lasting effects on adolescent girls' mental well-being, contributing to the development of mood disorders, PTSD, and self-harm behaviors.
- *Family dynamics:* Family dysfunction, parental mental illness, substance abuse within the family, and neglect or abuse can significantly affect adolescent mental health.
- *Cultural and socioeconomic factors:* Cultural expectations, socioeconomic status, access to mental health resources, and cultural attitudes toward seeking help can influence mental health outcomes.
- Pressures related to body image, appearance, academic performance, and social media can exacerbate stress and negatively impact self-image and mental health among adolescent girls.[4]

Addressing the mental health of young girls poses several challenges, stemming from societal, cultural, and systemic factors. They are often stigmatized, especially for young girls, leading to feelings of shame and reluctance to seek help. Cultural taboos surrounding mental illness can further exacerbate this stigma, hindering access to support and treatment. Young girls may face gender-specific pressures and expectations related to appearance, behavior, and academic performance, contributing to stress, anxiety, and low self-esteem.[5] Gender norms may also dictate how mental health concerns are perceived and addressed within families and communities.[6] Limited access to mental health services, including financial barriers, transportation challenges, and lack of culturally competent care, can prevent young girls from receiving timely and appropriate support. In many communities, there is a shortage of mental health professionals trained to address the specific needs of young girls.[4] The intersection of gender with other identities, such as race, ethnicity, sexuality, disability, or socioeconomic status, can compound the challenges young girls face in accessing mental health support. Marginalized girls may experience unique barriers and discrimination that impact their mental health outcomes. Mental health issues in young girls may go unrecognized or misdiagnosed due to gender biases in diagnostic criteria and clinical assessments. Symptoms of certain disorders, such as depression or ADHD, may present differently in girls compared to boys, leading to underdiagnosis and delayed intervention. Peer relationships and social dynamics can significantly influence the mental health of young girls. Bullying, social exclusion, and pressure to conform to unrealistic standards on social media can contribute to feelings of inadequacy, isolation, and anxiety.[3] Young girls may experience trauma, abuse, or adverse childhood experiences that impact their mental health and well-being. Addressing the underlying trauma and providing trauma-informed care is essential for effective mental health support. Lack of awareness about mental health issues among the general public and within educational and healthcare systems can impede early identification and intervention. Greater education and awareness are needed to promote understanding and reduce stigma surrounding girls' mental health.

STRATEGIES FOR SUPPORTING ADOLESCENT GIRLS' MENTAL HEALTH

It is important to recognize the signs and symptoms of these mental health issues early and provide them with the support, understanding, and access to professional help they need to thrive. Addressing these challenges requires a comprehensive approach that involves advocacy, education, policy reform, and community-based interventions.

Here are some strategies for effective management:

- *Early intervention:* Early detection and intervention are crucial for addressing mental health issues in young girls. Implementing screening programs in schools, primary care settings, and community organizations can help identify problems early and connect girls with appropriate support and treatment.

- *Accessible mental health services:* Ensure that mental health services are accessible and affordable for young girls, regardless of their socioeconomic status or geographical location. This may involve expanding mental health services in schools, offering teletherapy options, and providing financial assistance for families in need.
- *Culturally competent care:* Mental health services should be culturally sensitive and tailored to the diverse backgrounds and experiences of young girls. This includes providing language interpretation services, addressing cultural beliefs and practices, and involving family members in the treatment process when appropriate.
- *Holistic approach:* Take a holistic approach to mental health management that addresses the physical, emotional, social, and environmental factors influencing young girls' well-being. This may involve incorporating activities such as exercise, mindfulness, art therapy, and nutrition counseling into their treatment plans.
- *Psychoeducation:* Provide young girls and their families with psychoeducation about mental health issues, treatment options, and coping strategies. Empowering girls with knowledge about their condition can help reduce stigma, increase self-awareness, and promote active participation in their own care.[7]
- *Supportive environment:* Create a supportive environment at home, school, and in the community where young girls feel safe, valued, and supported. Foster positive relationships with peers, teachers, and mentors who can provide encouragement and guidance during difficult times.
- *Peer support groups:* Establish peer support groups or mentoring programs where young girls can connect with others who may be experiencing similar challenges. Peer support can provide validation, empathy, and practical advice for coping with mental health issues.
- *Collaboration and coordination:* Foster collaboration and coordination among mental health professionals, educators, healthcare providers, and community organizations involved in the care of young girls. This interdisciplinary approach ensures that girls receive comprehensive and coordinated support across different settings.
- *Empowerment and resilience-building:* Empower young girls to advocate for their own mental health needs and build resilience to cope with life's challenges. Encourage them to develop healthy coping skills, assertive communication, and problem-solving abilities that will serve them well into adulthood.

- *Prevention and education:* Invest in prevention programs and mental health education initiatives that promote positive mental health and well-being among young girls. Teach them skills for stress management, emotion regulation, and conflict resolution to prevent the onset of mental health problems.[8]

By implementing these strategies, we can effectively manage the mental health problems of young girls and support them in leading healthy, fulfilling lives.

ROLE OF GYNECOLOGIST IN ADDRESSING MENTAL HEALTH ISSUES OF ADOLESCENT GIRLS

Gynecologists play a significant role in addressing the mental health issues of adolescent girls, particularly those related to reproductive health and hormonal changes. Here is how:

- *Screening and awareness:* Gynecologists can screen adolescent girls for mental health issues during routine visits, such as annual check-ups or appointments related to contraception or menstrual health. They can ask about emotional well-being, stressors, and symptoms of common mental health disorders.
- *Addressing hormonal influences:* Hormonal changes during puberty, menstrual cycles, and reproductive health issues can impact mood and mental health. Gynecologists can educate girls about these hormonal fluctuations and how they may affect their emotions, providing reassurance and strategies for managing symptoms.[9]
- *Providing contraceptive counseling:* Adolescent girls may experience anxiety or depression related to concerns about contraception, unintended pregnancy, or sexual health. Gynecologists can offer confidential counseling, discuss contraceptive options, and address any emotional or psychological barriers to contraceptive use.
- *Referral to mental health professionals:* Gynecologists can identify signs of mental health issues and refer adolescent girls to mental health professionals, such as therapists, psychologists, or psychiatrists, for further evaluation and treatment.[3] They can collaborate with mental health providers to ensure comprehensive care.
- *Supporting patients with reproductive health concerns:* Adolescent girls with reproductive health concerns, such as polycystic ovary syndrome (PCOS), endometriosis, or menstrual disorders, may experience psychological distress related to their symptoms or diagnosis.[8] Gynecologists can offer support, validate their experiences, and connect them with resources for coping and managing their condition.
- *Promoting holistic well-being:* Gynecologists can promote holistic well-being by addressing not only physical health but also mental and

emotional health. They can encourage healthy lifestyle habits, stress management techniques, and self-care practices that support mental wellness.

By integrating mental health awareness and support into their practice, gynecologists can contribute to the overall well-being of adolescent girls and help address the complex interplay between reproductive health and mental health.[9]

CONCLUSION

Managing the mental health problems of young girls requires a multifaceted approach that addresses their unique needs and challenges. By addressing their unique needs and prioritizing their mental health and well-being, we can create a more supportive and inclusive environment where all girls have the opportunity to live happily.

By implementing targeted interventions that address their diverse needs, we can promote resilience, empowerment, and positive mental health outcomes among adolescent girls.

REFERENCES

1. Clayborne ZM, Varin M, Colman I. Systematic review and meta-analysis: adolescent depression and long-term psychosocial outcomes. J Am Acad Child Adolesc Psychiatry. 2019;58(1):72-9.
2. Cucchi A, Ryan D, Konstantakopoulos G, Stroumpa S, Kaçar AŞ, Renshaw S, et al. Lifetime prevalence of non-suicidal self-injury in patients with eating disorders: a systematic review and meta-analysis. Psychol Med. 2016;46(7):1345-58.
3. O'Reilly M, Dogra N, Whiteman N, Hughes J, Eruyar S, Reilly P. Is social media bad for mental health and wellbeing? Exploring the perspectives of adolescents. Clin Child Psychol Psychiatry. 2018;23:601-13.
4. Holland G, Tiggemann M. A systematic review of the impact of the use of social networking sites on body image and disordered eating outcomes. Body Image. 2016;17:100-10.
5. Karim F, Oyewande AA, Abdalla LF, Chaudhry Ehsanullah R, Khan S. Social media use and its connection to mental health: a systematic review. Cureus. 2020;12:0.
6. Hyde JS, Mezulis AH. Gender differences in depression: biological, affective, cognitive, and sociocultural factors. Harv Rev Psychiatr. 2020;28(1):4-13.
7. Plener PL, Schumacher TS, Munz LM, Groschwitz RC. The longitudinal course of non-suicidal self-injury and deliberate self-harm: a systematic review of the literature. Borderline personality disorder and emotion dysregulation. 2015;2(1):1-11.
8. Mehta N, Croudace T, Davies DSC. Public mental health: evidenced-based priorities. Lancet. 2015;385:1472-75.
9. 2022 National Healthcare Quality and Disparities Report [Internet]. Rockville (MD): Agency for Healthcare Research and Quality (US); 2022 Oct. Child and Adolescent Mental Health. Available from: https://www.ncbi.nlm.nih.gov/books/NBK587174/.

CHAPTER 23

Hysteroscopic Tubal Cannulation

Pratik Tambe, Suyesha Khanijao

INTRODUCTION

Infertility is defined as the inability to conceive after 1 year of unprotected intercourse. As per the World Health Organization (WHO) statistics released in October 2023, approximately one in six or 17.5% of the adult population faces infertility, which means that there is an urgent need for high-quality fertility care for those in need.

The new data shows almost no variation in the prevalence of infertility between regions. The rates are comparable for high-, middle-, and low-income countries, indicating that this is a major health challenge globally. Lifetime prevalence was 17.8% in high-income countries and 16.5% in low- and middle-income countries.[1]

Female infertility accounts for 40% of cases out of which up to 35% may be due to a tubal factor. In 10–25% of tubal obstruction, the localization of the narrowing is at the proximal end of the fallopian tube.

TUBAL INFERTILITY BASICS

In developed countries, the most common causes of infertility due to tubal occlusion are salpingitis due to chlamydia and other infections, salpingitis isthmica nodosa, endometriosis, and postsurgical adhesions. The narrowest part of the tube extends from the tubal ostium to the ampullary isthmic part, and thus, it is more prone to infections. Tubal damage owing to pelvic inflammatory disease (PID) is reported to be 12%, 23%, and 54% after one, two, and three episodes of PID, respectively.

Tubal obstruction can be temporary/false or true. A temporary proximal tubal obstruction can be due to mucous plugs, mechanical agglutination, or weak intraluminal microadhesions. The decision to operate and surgical resolution for the same needs to be made based on the type of obstruction, financial implications, expected success rate, age of the patient, and other concurrent associated reasons for infertility. With the easy availability, affordability, and accessibility of in vitro fertilization (IVF), tubal surgical procedures to restore patency are becoming less common in modern clinical practice.

ANATOMY OF THE PROXIMAL FALLOPIAN TUBE

The proximal tube is described in the surgical literature as the uterotubal junction (UTJ). It is defined as the part of the tube that marks the transition area between the intramural (interstitial) and isthmic portions. The diameter of the tubal lumen in the proximal 4–5 cm is 1 mm or less. The cornual portion of the uterus and tube is very vascular because of the network of vessels coursing through this area. The small caliber thick muscular wall and reduced proportion of ciliated cells in the epithelium of the proximal tube predispose this segment to blockage.[2]

The normal intramural oviduct ranges from 1.5 to 2.5 cm in length and takes a straight/curved course to the UTJ. It is 0.8–1.2 mm in diameter and can accommodate a cannula of 1.0–1.2 mm in diameter without epithelial damage. Each ostium is situated at the apex of the uterotubal gutter and can be seen hysteroscopically at the bottom of a saucer-shaped depression as a sharp membranous ring.

Therefore, if one passes a flexible smooth walled J-shaped directional cannula through the internal os and directs it toward the left or right, it will follow the uterotubal gutter toward the respective tubal ostium under vision. The knowledge of this anatomy helps us in designing instruments, planning the procedure, and negotiating through the blockage. **Figure 1** illustrates normal tubal anatomy.

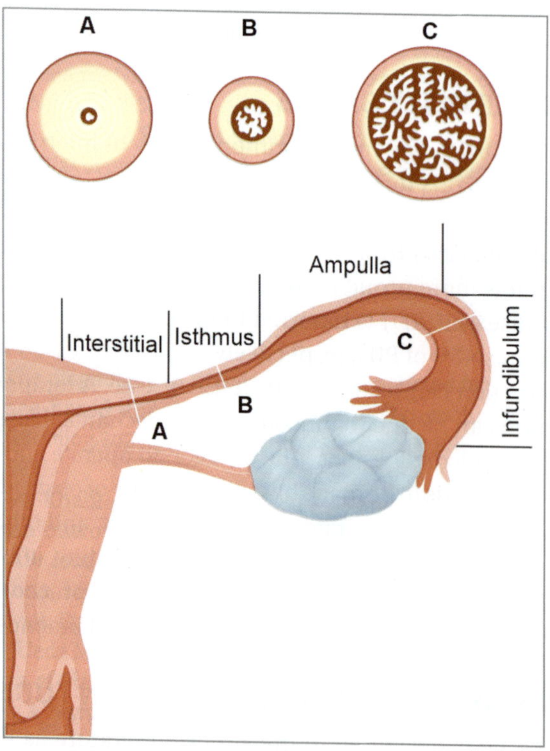

Fig. 1: Normal tubal anatomy with cross-section of lumen at various points.

DIAGNOSIS OF PROXIMAL TUBAL BLOCK

Proximal tubal obstruction has been classified into nodular (salpingitis isthmica nodosa or endometriosis), non-nodular (true fibrotic occlusion), and so-called "pseudo" occlusion (detritus, polyps, or hypoplastic tubes).

The proximal tubal damage can be diagnosed when there is failure of contrast medium to enter the intramural or isthmic portion of tube. The methods to diagnose it are by saline sonosalpingography, selective salpingography, hysterosalpingography (HSG) or by chromopertubation during laparoscopy.

The most commonly done test for diagnosis of proximal tubal occlusion (PTO) traditionally is HSG. The disadvantage is that it cannot differentiate between true blockage and muscular spasm. The false positive rate may be as high as 25%. Excessive pressure while pushing of dye can also cause false occlusion. The confirmation of PTO can be done with laparoscopy and chromopertubation, repeat HSG under analgesic cover, or salpingography.

TUBAL CANNULATION PROCEDURES

Tubal cannulation is the process of accessing the interior of the fallopian tubes and relieving any obstruction within. It is a highly specialized technique which requires a combined hysteroscopy and laparoscopy for optimum results. This intricate process involves navigating the narrow and winding anatomy of the fallopian tubes, often in the presence of obstructions or anatomical variations.

Successful tubal cannulation is crucial for various diagnostic and therapeutic interventions, such as the assessment of tubal patency, the treatment of tubal blockages, and the facilitation of embryo transfer during IVF procedures. Careful preprocedure planning and couple counseling, the use of specialized instruments, and a good understanding of pelvic and tubal anatomy are essential for surgeons to safely and effectively perform this challenging procedure.

Techniques such as the use of flexible hysteroscopes, the application of selective tubal cannulation, and the employment of ancillary tools such as guidewires and catheters can enhance the clinician's ability to navigate the fallopian tubes and achieve the desired clinical outcomes.

METHODS OF CANNULATION

The procedures described for proximal tubal cannulation include:

- Flexible guidewire via hysteroscopy
- Falloposcopic-guided cannulation
- Transcervical balloon cannulation with linear catheter
- Under fluoroscopy control

Flexible Guidewire via Hysteroscopy

This is the most commonly performed of all the methods for tubal cannulation.

A 2.9-mm 30° telescope (hysteroscope) with a 5-mm continuous flow operative sheath is used along with a Novy cornual cannulation set containing a J-shaped 3-Fr catheter with a guidewire within it **(Fig. 2)**. The catheter is introduced through the operative channel up to the tubal ostium of blocked tubes under hysteroscopic guidance. Selective chromopertubation is performed under laparoscopic control to confirm the presence of a block and may relieve pseudo-obstruction.

The guidewire provides strength and rigidity so that the catheter can be controlled for the procedure. The catheter with the guidewire is then introduced for 1–2 cm to overcome the proximal tubal obstruction. The methylene blue dye is then reintroduced, and tubal patency is observed under laparoscopic guidance.

Falloposcopic Cannulation

A specialized falloscope which is a thin, flexible endoscope is carefully inserted through the incision and guided into the fallopian tube under direct visualization from the fimbrial end of the fallopian tube. The falloscope allows for the evaluation of the tubal lumen and the identification of any obstructions or lesions. Therapeutic interventions such as tubal cannulation or adhesiolysis can then be performed as needed. This is an extremely technical and sophisticated procedure, which is not commonly being performed today.

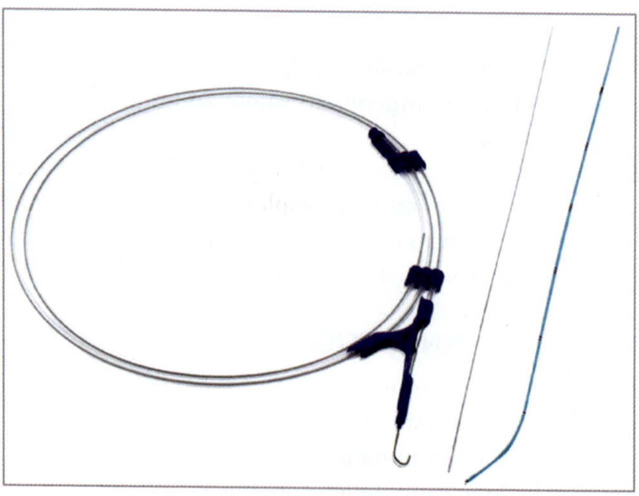

Fig. 2: Novy cornual cannulation set with flexible J-shaped sheath and guidewire.

Fluoroscopy Control

A 21-Fr hysteroscope is inserted into the uterine cavity using normal saline as the distending media. Tubal cannulation is performed with a Novy catheter. The outer catheter and metal stylet are then inserted into the visualized ostium of the occluded fallopian tube.

Once inserted, the C-arm is brought to the pelvic region, and an initial single-shot imaging is used to confirm appropriate location. At this point, injection of contrast dye is performed under real-time fluoroscopic imaging. If no fill of the fallopian tube is seen, then a 3-Fr inner catheter with a 2-Fr inner guidewire is snaked through the initial outer catheter and is probed laterally into the intramural and isthmic portions of the fallopian tube.

Repeat contrast injection is performed, and images are saved and reviewed following the completion of the procedure. In essence, the procedure is similar but does not utilize laparoscopy and may be performed as an office procedure with local anesthesia and mild sedation with appropriate counseling.

SUCCESS RATES

These will vary depending on the cause of the block, duration of infertility, and operator expertise. A study from India where 66 women showed bilateral tubal block on HSG was able to achieve tubal patency following hysteroscopic tubal cannulation in 89% of women. The clinical pregnancy rate within 6 months after the procedure was 27%.[3]

Another study on 168 women included 107 (63.7%) with bilateral proximal obstruction and 61 (36.3%) with unilateral obstruction. The successful recanalization rate was 54.2% per tube and 61.9% per patient. In the 93 patients in whom at least 1 fallopian tube was successfully recanalized, 43% spontaneous pregnancies occurred within 24 months, of which 37.6% were intrauterine pregnancies and 30.1% resulted in live births. Patients with unilateral obstruction in whom cannulation was successful had the highest clinical pregnancy rates of 60.7% at 2 years.[4]

A study from New York included 32 women who underwent fluoroscopically guided hysteroscopic tubal cannulation (FHTC). Of those women with bilateral obstruction, 100% of subjects achieved at least unilateral patency, while patency was achieved in 88.5% subjects with unilateral obstruction.

A total of 90.6% women had at least unilateral successful cannulation with 89.5% of proximally obstructed tubes opened. Asymptomatic tubal perforation occurred in one case. Of the participants, 34.5% achieved intrauterine pregnancies without IVF in an average of 65 days from the procedure. There were no multiple pregnancies and one ectopic pregnancy.[5]

PROCEDURAL CHALLENGES

While hysteroscopic cannulation is a valuable diagnostic and therapeutic tool, it is not without its challenges. One of the primary challenges is the complex anatomy of the female reproductive system, which can make it difficult to access certain areas, such as the uterine cornua or the fallopian tubes.

Additionally, some patients may have preexisting conditions, such as cervical stenosis or uterine scarring, which can further complicate the procedure. The existence of tubal adhesions and scarring need to be confirmed laparoscopically to ensure that the lateral two-thirds of the tubes are healthy. Distortion of the anatomy and change in the location of the ostia should raise a suspicion of existing pelvic adhesions distorting the tubal anatomy, in which case proximal tubal cannulation would be reduced to a surgical exercise without improving the patient's fertility.

Another challenge is ensuring patient comfort and safety throughout the procedure. Hysteroscopic cannulation can be uncomfortable for some patients, and there is a risk of complications, such as uterine perforation or bleeding. Careful patient preparation, the use of general anesthesia, and the expertise of the healthcare provider are all critical in mitigating these risks and ensuring a successful outcome.

COMPLICATIONS

These occur in about 6% of cases. As described earlier, careful preoperative assessment, case selection, couple counseling, and ensuring simultaneous laparoscopic visualization with two camera systems will go a long way to reducing the incidence of complications. **Table 1** lists the common complications encountered during the procedure.

TABLE 1: Complications of hysteroscopic tubal cannulation.

Complication	*Description*	*Management*
Uterine perforation	Hysteroscope or instrument pushed through uterine wall	Immediate surgical intervention
Cervical laceration	Tearing of the cervix during cannulation	Suturing or medical management
Excessive bleeding	Significant bleeding during or after the procedure	Medication, compression, or surgical intervention
Infection	Bacterial or viral infection of the uterus or surrounding tissues	Antibiotic treatment
Fluid overload	Excess fluid absorption during the procedure	Medication, monitoring, and fluid management

CONCLUSION

The most common treatment offered to the patients of tubal block is IVF, which is more easily available and accessible compared to a few years ago. There is enough evidence available to support the role of salpingography and proximal tubal cannulation in opening the block and restoring fertility in patients who present with an isolated proximal block. The vast majority of patients may have a reversible obstruction, which may not require extensive fertility enhancing endoscopic surgery or IVF.[6]

The success of the procedure depends on a variety of factors including the type of block, the expertise of the surgeon, and the utilization of simultaneous laparoscopic control. The role of fluoroscopic tubal catheterization is one more option now available in our armamentarium for proximal tubal patency.

REFERENCES

1. World Health Organization. (2023). Infertility Prevalence Estimates, 1990–2021. [online] Available from https://www.who.int/publications-detail-redirect/978920068315 [Last accessed September, 2024].
2. Roberts A. Fallopian tube recanalization for the management of infertility. CVIR Endovasc. 2023;6:13.
3. Banerjee K, Singla B. Novel use of hysteroscopy in the assessment of tubal patency in difficult cannulation. Gynecol Minim Invasive Ther. 2021;10(3):166-7.
4. Hou HY, Chen YQ, Li TC, Hu CX, Chen X, Yang ZH. Outcome of laparoscopy-guided hysteroscopic tubal catheterization for infertility due to proximal tubal obstruction. J Minim Invasive Gynecol. 2014;21(2):272-8.
5. Keltz M, Brown EC, Frishman GN, Sauerbrun-Cutler MT. Fluoroscopically-guided hysteroscopic tubal cannulation: a procedure for proximal tubal obstruction. JSLS. 2022;26(4):e2022.00047.
6. Soliman AT, Salem HA. Evaluation of hysteroscopic tubal cannulation under laparoscopic control versus intracytoplasmic sperm injection in cases with proximal tubal obstruction. EBWHJ. 2013;3(3):147-53.

CHAPTER 24

Placenta Accreta Spectrum Disorders

Kanchan Prasad, Pratik Tambe

INTRODUCTION

Placenta accreta spectrum (PAS) disorders is an umbrella term for a variety of pregnancy complications due to abnormal placental implantation, which traditionally includes placenta accreta, increta, and percreta. Over a period of time, especially during the past couple of decades, the prevalence of PAS has increased, and the clinical importance of these conditions is significant, because they represent a risk to life and owing to the severity of the complications they present with.[1]

The underlying pathology is a focal or diffuse pathological adherence of the placenta to the myometrium due to abnormal trophoblast invasion. The placenta fails to separate spontaneously after delivery and cannot be forcibly separated without causing catastrophic obstetric hemorrhage. As described earlier, the complications include severe maternal morbidity with increased risk of blood transfusion, sepsis, coagulopathy, intensive care unit admission, operative injury to the urinary tract, and cesarean/obstetric hysterectomy with consequent loss of fertility.[2,3]

EPIDEMIOLOGY

Placenta accreta spectrum was first reported by Irving et al. in 1927 with an incidence of 0.12 in 1,000 women. The rate of PAS has increased over time with reported incidence between 1 in 2,510 (1970s) and 1 in 4,017 (1980s). It was reported as 1 in 533 between 1982 and 2002. This increasing rate is linked to increased rate of cesarean delivery, a known risk factor for PAS. The main risk factors for PAS are previous cesarean delivery and placenta previa. In women with placenta previa, the risk of PAS is 3%, 11%, 40%, 61%, and 67%, after 1, 2, 3, 4, 5, or more cesarean deliveries.[4,5]

ANTENATAL SCREENING AND DIAGNOSIS (BOX 1)

Placenta accreta spectrum remains undetected before delivery in around 50% of cases, but diagnostic accuracy can be up to 95% in good tertiary care institutions. This is owing to the findings that are subjective in nature and depend on the expertise of the clinician. The early detection of PAS disorders is of clinical significance as it alerts the obstetric team to anticipate the probability

BOX 1: Whom to prioritize for screening?

- History of previous damage to the uterus
- Superficial uterine cavity injury, e.g., curettage, radiation, endometritis, endometrial ablation, Asherman's syndrome, endometrial resection, manual removal of the placenta, uterine-artery embolization, and myomectomy
- Full thickness uterine wall injury, e.g., surgical incision, perforation, or previous uterine rupture
- *Other risk factors:* In vitro fertilization (IVF) pregnancy, multifetal gestation, advanced maternal age, high parity, and placenta accreta spectrum (PAS) in a previous pregnancy

of significant maternal morbidity. Accurate assessment of risk is crucial for avoiding false positive diagnoses, as in 98% of low-risk pregnancies with normal placental placement, two or more imaging signs of PAS may be present.[6,7]

Timing of Screening[8]

- *First trimester:* Cesarean scar pregnancy is a precursor to PAS disorders and can be detected as early as 6–10 weeks.
- *Second trimester:* It is ideally performed at 18–24 weeks along with the anomaly scan; a repeat evaluation at 32 weeks is recommended.

Diagnostic Modalities for Screening Approaches[9]

Two-dimensional (2D) grayscale and color Doppler imaging remain the cornerstone of prenatal PAS diagnosis, with magnetic resonance imaging (MRI) serving as a supplementary tool in select cases to enhance diagnostic accuracy and inform clinical decision-making.

A few key points to consider during ultrasound diagnosis:

- Transabdominal scans are commonly used to diagnose PAS, but a transvaginal approach is more effective for patients with high body mass index (BMI) and for focusing on the leading placental edge, lower uterine wall, bladder interface, cervical canal, and internal os. Transabdominal scans can be improved by selecting a higher frequency (5–9 MHz) transducer or linear probe.
- Examination should be carried out on a full bladder; without a full bladder, signs such as bladder wall interruption, placental bulge, and uterovesical hypervascularity cannot be appropriately assessed. Excessive probe pressure should be avoided during transabdominal scanning, because it can cause an apparent loss of the retroplacental clear zone.

Ultrasound Signs[10]

- *Neovascularization:* It develops at the level of the serosal surface of the uterus or within the uterovesical fold of the peritoneum in the case of a low-lying or previa placenta.
- *Bridging vessels and bladder wall interruption:* On grayscale imaging in an anterior low-lying placenta, it may appear as pairs of hyperechoic lines (the "=" sign) parallel to the uterine serosa and posterior bladder wall. This sign is commonly referred to as "bladder wall interruption" in grayscale ultrasound and bridging vessels in color Doppler imaging. Bridging vessels are the most important sign, because they only appear when there is an abundance of neovascularity on the serosal surface.
- *Subplacental hypervascularity:* PAS causes hypervascularity on the serosal surface rather than within the myometrium itself. Adenomyosis is distinguished from PAS by its thick cystic and vascular myometrium, whereas PAS has an abnormally thin myometrium.
- *Myometrial invasion and abnormal lacunae:* Abnormal lacunae are the most common ultrasound signs of PAS. Lacunae are large, irregular anechoic, or hypoechoic areas in the placenta that give it a "moth-eaten" appearance. Placental lakes, which contain slow-moving blood, can be easily compressed with an ultrasound probe, while typical PAS-related lacunae cannot. PAS-related lacunae are frequently found in the region of abnormal placentation, while lakes are typically sparse and widely distributed. Placental infarctions, characterized by hypoechoic regions and hyperechogenic rims, are frequently linked to pre-eclampsia and restricted fetal growth and should be differentiated from lacunes or lakes with a hyperechogenic rim.
- On color Doppler, PAS-related lacunae are typically confirmed by demonstrating high-velocity flow (>10 cm/s) with feeder vessels, while lakes can have very low flow velocity, for which signals are rarely detected on Doppler. Echogenic cystic lesions caused by placental infarctions have no flow on color Doppler.
- *Deficiency of Nitabuch's layer:* This causes subsequent "fusion" of placenta and myometrium.
- *Loss of retroplacental clear zone:* The echolucent space between the placenta and endometrium is known as the retroplacental hypoechoic zone. The loss of this zone signifies the fusion of the placenta and myometrium.
- *Myometrial thinning:* Myometrial thickness <1 mm behind the placenta has been reported as a sign of PAS. A "uterine window" can occur when the placenta overlies a simple uterine scar dehiscence without abnormal placentation. The presence or absence of additional sonographic and clinical PAS markers will distinguish between the two pathologies.

- *Placental bulge:* Inadequate residual myometrium to maintain the structural integrity of the uterus causes outpouching of the placenta known as a placental bulge. The dehiscence of a uterine scar with normal placentation can result in the same picture. However, in these cases, the bulge is usually smaller, and the placenta is homogeneous without evidence of other imaging signs of PAS.

The International Federation of Gynecology and Obstetrics Guidelines 2019 (Table 1)

The International Society for Placenta Accreta Spectrum [formerly known as European Working Group on Abnormally Invasive Placenta (AIP)] proposed a standardized definition of the PAS ultrasound descriptors in 2016, in order to increase the diagnostic accuracy, and to facilitate the international collaboration. This standardized terminology has been subsequently incorporated into the International Federation of Gynecology and Obstetrics (FIGO) 2019 guidelines on the prenatal diagnosis and screening of PAS.[9,11]

Magnetic Resonance Imaging (Box 2)[12]

Magnetic resonance imaging has been recommended as a second-line imaging tool for the diagnosis of PAS to assess the depth of invasion and the lateral extension of myometrial invasion, especially with posterior placentation and in women with ultrasound suspicion of parametrial invasion and in high maternal BMI. The International Society for Placenta Accreta Spectrum (formerly EW-AIP) has proposed MRI descriptors of PAS to facilitate international collaboration.

Representative images of the ultrasound and MRI findings are presented in **Figures 1 to 5**.

Biomarkers

Several potential biomarkers have been studied in PAS, showing variability of measurement depending on gestational age. The beta-subunit of human chorionic gonadotropin (β-hCG) has been shown to be lower and pregnancy-associated plasma protein A (PAPP-A) higher at 11–12 weeks of gestation in the serum of women with PAS disorders. Serum β-hCG and alpha-fetoprotein (AFP) levels are higher in cases of PAS at 14–22 weeks. Currently, there is no evidence of an effective biomarker for serological screening of PAS.[9]

TABLE 1: Unified descriptors [European Working Group on Abnormally Invasive Placenta (EW-AIP)] for ultrasound findings in placenta accreta spectrum (PAS) disorders.

Descriptor/ultrasound findings	***Definitions***
2D grayscale imaging:	
Loss of the "clear zone"	Loss of the hypoechoic plane in the myometrium underneath the placental bed
Abnormal placental lacunae	Presence of numerous lacunae including some that are large and irregular often containing turbulent flow in grayscale imaging
Bladder wall interruption	Loss or interruption of the bright bladder wall (the hyperechoic band or "line" between the uterine serosa and the bladder lumen)
Myometrial thinning	Thinning of the myometrium overlying the placenta to <1 mm or undetectable
Placental bulge	Deviation of the uterine serosa away from the expected plane, caused by an abnormal bulge of placental tissue into a neighboring organ, typically the bladder
Focal exophytic mass	Placental tissue is seen breaking through the uterine serosa and extending beyond it. Most often seen inside a filled urinary bladder
Color Doppler imaging:	
Uterovesical hypervascularity	Striking amount of color Doppler signal seen between the myometrium and the posterior wall of the bladder
Subplacental hypervascularity	Striking amount of color Doppler signal seen in the placental bed
Bridging vessels	Vessels appearing to extend from the placenta across the myometrium and beyond the serosa into the bladder or other organs. Often running perpendicular to the myometrium
Placental lacunae feeder vessels	Vessels with high-velocity blood flow, leading from the myometrium into the placental lacunae, causing turbulence upon entry
3D intraplacental hypervascularity	Complex, irregular arrangement of numerous placental vessels, exhibiting tortuous courses and varying calibers

BOX 2: MRI findings in placenta accreta spectrum (PAS).

- Heterogeneous placenta
- Placental bulge
- Dark intraplacental bands
- Placental ischemic infarction
- Loss of retroplacental dark zone
- Myometrial thinning
- Bladder wall interruption
- Focal exophytic mass
- Abnormal vascularization of the placental bed

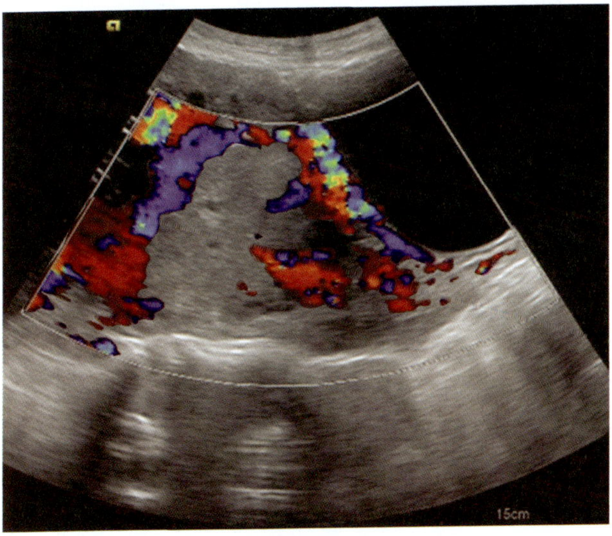

Fig. 1: Subplacental hypervascularity.

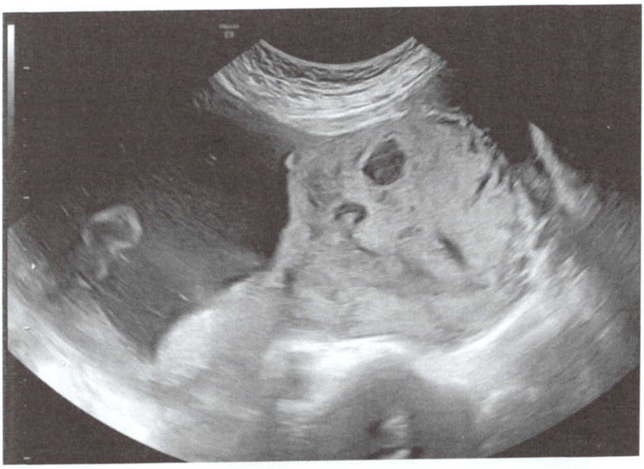

Fig. 2: Multiple lacunae.

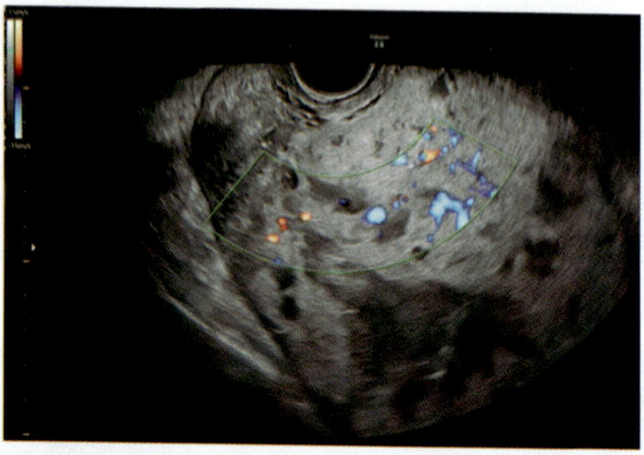

Fig. 3: Multiple lacunae with increased color flow within.

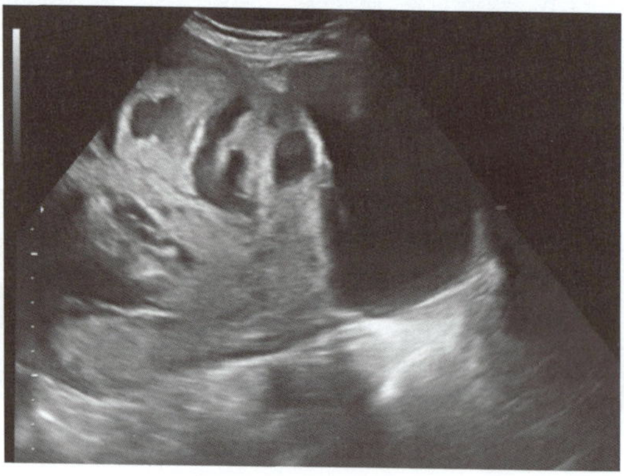

Fig. 4: Thinned-out myometrium with the obliterated retroplacental clear zone.

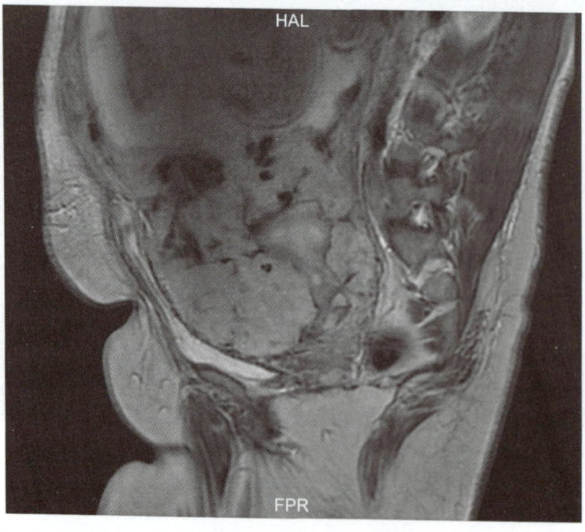

Fig. 5: Intraplacental dark bands with thinned-out myometrium.

NEW PAS CLASSIFICATION FIGO 2020 (TABLE 2)

A panel of experts in 2020 proposed a new pathological classification for PAS disorders, which was endorsed by FIGO.

MANAGEMENT PRINCIPLES

Placenta accreta spectrum disorders pose significant risks, including obstetric hemorrhage, urological injury, intensive care unit admission coagulopathy, multisystem organ failure, and even maternal mortality. Surgical risks rise with the extent of placental invasion. Accurate antenatal diagnosis, diligent delivery planning, and complication management by a multidisciplinary excellence care team are critical for reducing maternal morbidity and mortality.

DELIVERY CONSIDERATIONS

A planned delivery in a center of excellence with a dedicated multidisciplinary team is highly recommended. Ensure access to blood products, surgical expertise in complex pelvic surgery, intensive care facilities, and obstetric anesthetists. The optimum time for scheduled delivery is controversial.

For a stable patient with no antepartum hemorrhage, preterm premature rupture of membranes (PPROM), or preterm labor, planned delivery between 34+0 and 35+6 weeks of gestation is recommended by the American College of Obstetricians and Gynecologists (ACOG) and at 36–37 weeks by FIGO. The risk of hemorrhage and the risk of preterm should be weighed. With episodes of antepartum hemorrhage, PPROM, and contractions, planned preterm delivery is warranted.[4,14]

A brief management for PAS disorders is presented in **Flowchart 1** as a detailed description of the operative management is beyond the scope of this chapter.

CONCLUSION

Placenta accreta spectrum disorders pose a high risk of hemorrhage, surgical complications, and maternal mortality. Given the global trend of increasing cesarean section rates, the incidence of PAS is likely to rise further in the future. The preliminary diagnostic approach for risk triage involves a clinical risk assessment, including a history of uterine surgery and a thorough ultrasound of the placenta.

For antenatally diagnosed cases, cesarean hysterectomy is the most common and definitive treatment option. The institution's expertise and resources, the severity of PAS, and the patient's preferences all influence whether conservative or alternative management approaches are used. Furthermore, a multidisciplinary team of experienced obstetricians, radiologists, and histopathologists should be involved in establishing a definitive diagnosis of PAS. Future research should focus on providing the best screening, diagnosis, and treatment options for women suffering from PAS disorders.

TABLE 2: New pathological classification endorsed by FIGO.[13]

Historical classification	*Clinical classification*	*Description*	*Pathological classification*	*Description*
Abnormal adherent placenta (placenta adherenta or creta)	Grade 1	• *At vaginal delivery:* No separation with synthetic oxytocin and gently controlled cord traction unable to manually develop a clean plane of separation between placenta and myometrium; often requires curettage • *If laparotomy is required:* No placental tissue is seen invading through the surface of the uterus, and there is no or minimal neovascularity	Grade 1	Areas of absent decidua between villi and myometrium; uniform myometrial thickness without thinning
Abnormally invasive placentation (placenta increta)	Grade 2	• *At laparotomy:* – Abnormal macroscopic findings over the placental bed: bluish/purple coloring, distension called placental bulge – Significant amounts of hypervascularity – Dimple sign, with uterus pulling in – On gentle cord traction	Grade 2	Irregular placenta-myometrium interface, without involvement of outer myometrium (<75% of myometrial thickness); intact uterine serosa
Abnormally invasive placentation (placenta percreta)	Grade 3		Grade 3	

Contd...

Contd...

Historical classification	***Clinical classification***	***Description***	***Pathological classification***	***Description***
	Grade 3a: Limited to the uterine serosa	• *At laparotomy*: – Abnormal macroscopic findings on uterine surface Grade 2 and placental tissue seen through the surface of the uterus without extension to other organs – Placenta visible through extremely thin myometrium or single layer of serosa – A clear surgical plane can be identified between the bladder and uterus	Grade 3A	Irregular placenta-myometrium interface, placental involvement of outer myometrium (>75% thickness); intact uterine serosa (A = abnormal invasion)
Percreta	*Grade 3b:* With urinary bladder invasion	• *At laparotomy*: – Same as Grade 3a – Placental villi are seen to be invading into the bladder but no other organs – Clear surgical plane cannot be identified between the bladder and uterus	Grade 3D	Deep myometrial invasion with disruption of serosal surface (D = deep invasion)
Percreta	*Grade 3c:* With the invasion of other pelvic tissue/organs	• *At laparotomy:* – Same as Grade 3a – Placental villi are seen to be invading the broad ligament, vaginal wall, pelvic sidewall, or any other pelvic organ (with or without invasion of the bladder)	Grade 3E	Extrauterine extension with placental invasion into, or fibroadipose tissue extension to, extrauterine structures (E = extrauterine invasion)

Flowchart 1: Management for PAS disorders.[1]

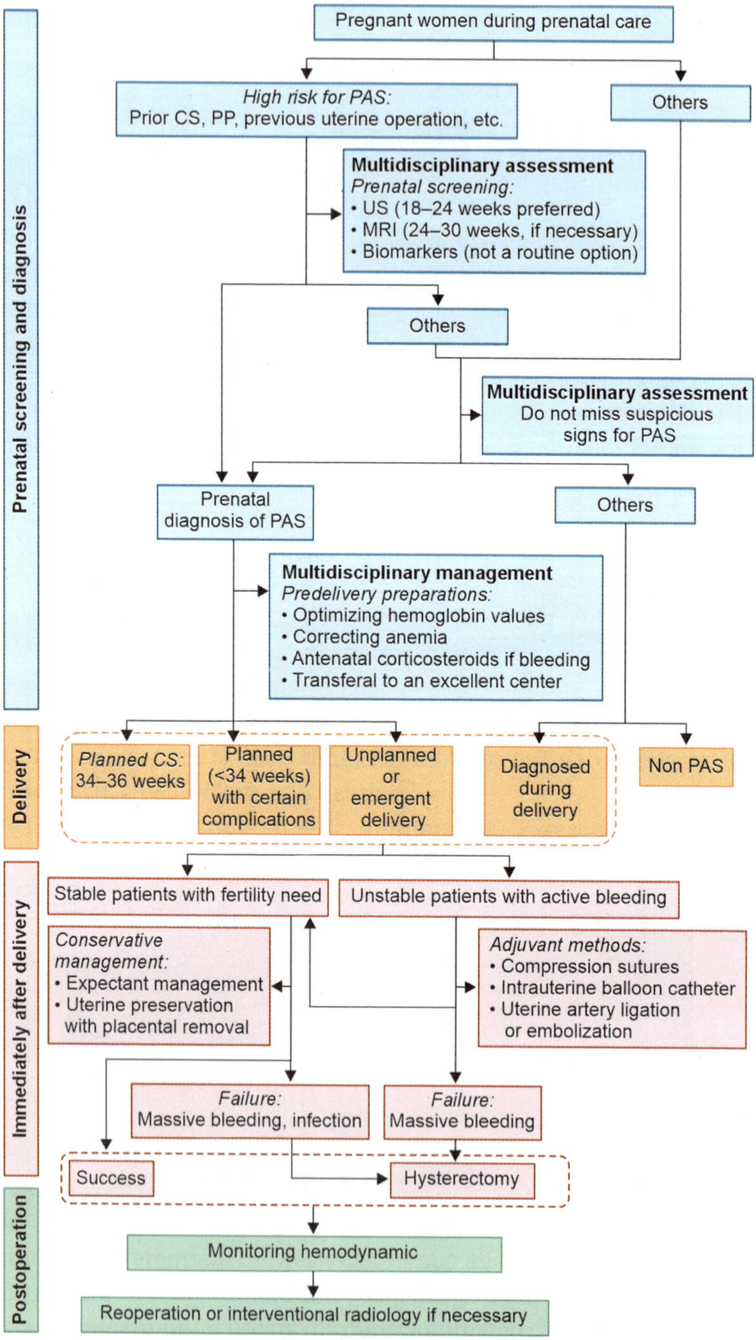

(CS: cesarean section; MRI: magnetic resonance imaging; PAS: placenta accreta spectrum; PP: placenta previa)

REFERENCES

1. Liu X, Wang Y, Wu Y, Zeng J, Yuan X, Tong C, et al. What we know about placenta accreta spectrum (PAS)? Eur J Obstet Gynecol Reprod Biol. 2021;259:81-9.
2. Morlando M, Collins S. Placenta accreta spectrum disorders: challenges, risks, and management strategies. Int J Women's Health. 2020;12:1033-45.
3. Morlando M, Schwickert A, Stefanovic V, Gziri MM, Pateisky P, Chalubinski KM, et al. Maternal and neonatal outcomes in planned versus emergency cesarean delivery for placenta accreta spectrum: a multinational database study. Acta Obstet Gynecol Scand. 2021;100:41-9.
4. American College of Obstetricians and Gynecologists. Placenta accreta spectrum. Obstetric Care Consensus No. 7. Obs Gynecol. 2018;132:e259-75.
5. Silver RM, Landon MB, Rouse DJ, Leveno KJ, Spong CY, Thom EA, et al. Maternal morbidity associated with multiple repeat cesarean deliveries. Obstet Gynecol. 2006;107(6):1226-32.
6. Jauniaux E, Bhide A. Prenatal ultrasound diagnosis and outcome of placenta previa accreta after cesarean delivery: a systematic review and meta-analysis. Am J Obstet Gynecol. 2017;217(1):27-36.
7. Philips J, Gurganus M, DeShields S, Cunningham T, Sinkovskaya E, Kanaan C, et al. Prevalence of sonographic markers of placenta accreta spectrum in low-risk pregnancies. Am J Perinatol. 2019;36:733-80.
8. Shazly SA, Hortu I, Shih J-C, Melekoglu R, Fan S, Ahmed FUA, et al. Prediction of clinical outcomes in women with placenta accreta spectrum using machine learning models: an international multicenter study. J Matern Fetal Neonatal Med. 2022;35(25):6644-53.
9. Jauniaux E, Bhide A, Kennedy A, Woodward P, Hubinont C, Collins S; FIGO Placenta Accreta Diagnosis and Management Expert Consensus Panel. FIGO consensus guidelines on placenta accreta spectrum disorders: prenatal diagnosis and screening. Int J Gynaecol Obstet. 2018;140(3):274-80.
10. Adu-Bredu TK, Owusu-Bempah A, Collins S. Accurate prenatal discrimination of placenta accreta spectrum from uterine dehiscence is necessary to ensure optimal management. BMJ Case Rep. 2021;14:e244286.
11. Collins SL, Ashcroft A, Braun T, Calda P, Langhoff-Roos J, Morel O, et al. Proposal for standardized ultrasound descriptors of abnormally invasive placenta (AIP). Ultrasound Obstet Gynecol. 2016;47:271-5.
12. Morel O, Collins SL, Uzan-Augui J, Masselli G, Duan J, Chabot-Lecoanet A-C, et al. A proposal for standardized magnetic resonance imaging (MRI) descriptors of abnormally invasive placenta (AIP): From the International Society for AIP. Diagn Interv Imaging. 2019;100(6):319-25.
13. Hecht JL, Baergen R, Ernst LM, Katzman PJ, Jacques SM, Jauniaux E, et al. Classification and reporting guidelines for the pathology diagnosis of placenta accreta spectrum (PAS) disorders: recommendations from an expert panel. Mod Pathol. 2020;33:2382-96.
14. Allen L, Jauniaux E, Hobson S, Papillon-Smith J, Belfort MA; FIGO Placenta Accreta Diagnosis and Management Expert Consensus Panel. FIGO consensus guidelines on placenta accreta spectrum disorders: Nonconservative surgical management. Int J Gynaecol Obstet. 2018;140(3):281-90.

Index

Page numbers followed by *b* refer to box, *f* refer to figure, *fc* refer to flowchart, and *t* refer to table.

D

E

F

G

H

I

T